Spring Forest Qigong Level One Manual

W9-CKB-030

Printed in the United States of America
Seventh Printing – January 2011

Notice: This manual and all Spring Forest Qigong teaching and learning materials are intended for your education of healthful practices. This manual and the other learning materials are not intended as a replacement for any medical treatment or therapy by a physician or other licensed health care provider. Rather, this manual and the other learning materials are intended to help you broaden your understanding of health and wellness and help you make informed choices of health options. Any application of the information in this manual and the other learning materials is at the student's discretion and sole responsibility.

ISBN 0–9740944–7–1

Cover design by Pixel Farms

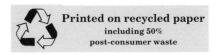

Printed on recycled paper
including 50%
post-consumer waste

Table of Contents

Table of Contents

Table of Contents

Biography

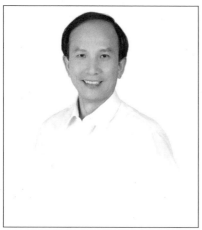

Chunyi Lin is a certified international Qigong Master and founder of Spring Forest Qigong. His fluency in numerous Chinese dialects provided him the rare opportunity to study with many of the most respected Qigong Masters in his native China. He has been teaching Qigong and using Qigong techniques to help others for more than twenty-five years. Master Lin is also highly skilled in Tai Chi, Chinese herbal medicine and acupuncture.

Lin is the founder and chairman of the Spring Forest Center in Eden Prairie, MN. As many as 10,000 people, from across the United States and many foreign countries, come to his center for healing assistance every year.

During 2004 he created an Educational Partnership with Normandale Community College of Bloomington, MN to provide fully accredited courses in Spring Forest Qigong health and healing techniques. All of the course curricula were created by Mr. Lin and he serves as the program director and lead instructor.

Lin was formerly a college professor in the Guangdon Province in China. In January of 2005, he was awarded a Masters Degree in Human Development-Holistic Health & Wellness from St. Mary's University in Minneapolis, MN. Lin served as Director of Qigong Programs at Anoka-Ramsey Community College in Anoka,

Minnesota, from 1999 to 2004.

Lin teaches four levels of Spring Forest Qigong and has created a series of home learning materials for students, including DVD's, guided audio meditations and reference manuals. Master Lin's vision is "a healer in every family and a world without pain". He is a frequent keynote speaker at national health conferences.

He is coauthor of a #1 Amazon.com bestseller, Born A Healer, and coauthor with Dr. Nisha Manek of the Mayo Clinic of a chapter on qigong in the recently released Textbook of Complementary and Alternative Medicine, 2nd Edition. Lin is also a member of the Transformational Leadership Council founded by Jack Canfield.

Since coming to the United States in 1995, he has helped over 100,000 people learn about the powerful, healing benefits of Spring Forest Qigong. He now devotes all of his time to the teaching of Spring Forest Qigong and helping others.

He lives in the Twin Cities with his family.

Learn more about Master Lin, his vision and Spring Forest Qigong by visiting the web at: www.springforestqigong.com.

Welcome

Hello, my dear friend:

Welcome to Spring Forest Qigong. Each and every one of us is born with the ability to help ourselves and others to heal, physically, mentally, emotionally and spiritually. This is the simple, yet powerful and wonderful message of Spring Forest Qigong.

This manual opens a door for you to begin to experience the profoundly simple and powerful healing art of Spring Forest Qigong. When you read this manual you will find my energy and the love energy of the universe with you. It is my hope that as you learn and practice Spring Forest Qigong you will come to experience that "You were born a healer" and along with that the greatest joy possible.

Why "Spring Forest" Qigong?

The name Spring Forest Qigong is very meaningful. Imagine a forest in springtime. Spring is the season of awakening from the cold, dormant period of winter, a time of new life and rebirth. A forest is a beautiful place with trees, other plants and many animals, a natural haven where diverse living things thrive in harmony.

However, one tree does not make a forest. A forest is alive with many, many trees. This is how I see Spring Forest Qigong. It offers everyone a simple yet very powerful way to awaken their natural healing ability. But it is not just one way, one tree standing alone. Spring Forest Qigong works in harmony with other practitioners of all kinds who use their techniques to help people to become free of pain and sickness and to live the richest, most rewarding life possible.

Learning Level One

Throughout this manual you will find the exercises and meditations of Spring Forest Qigong Level One. Each exercise includes a section that describes the purpose of that movement or meditation, the benefit you can receive and a detailed description so you can get started right away.

You will also learn *"swordfingers"*, a simple yet powerful healing technique that you can use to help others to heal. You can even use this technique to help yourself!

To assist you in learning Level One we have created additional learning materials. We offer a DVD which guides you through the active exercises of Level One step-by-step. All you need to do is follow along. There are also CD's with both guided meditations and meditation music that are very beneficial, enjoyable and helpful in learning Spring Forest Qigong. If you are interested in practicing Spring Forest Qigong we highly recommend these other learning resources.

Before we begin with specific Spring Forest Qigong exercises and meditations let's explore:

- Energy and the Miracle of Qigong
- How Qigong Works
- What is Spring Forest Qigong
- The Rewards and Benefits of Spring Forest Qigong
- The Question of Religion and Qigong

Energy and the Miracle of Qigong

Everything in the universe is energy. Since the work of Albert Einstein, physicists have recognized that our world, indeed the entire universe, is composed of dynamic relationships of energy.

Everything from an inanimate rock or a stream to a living being is formed of energy. Energy cannot be created, it cannot be destroyed, but it can be transformed.

Qigong is a study of energy and since everything is a form of energy qigong is a study of the whole universe, including physics, chemistry, psychology, biology, astrology, electricity and medicine. In China, the ancient art of qigong has been practiced for many different purposes for thousands of years and the benefits of qigong are as many as there are aspects to life. In fact there are thousands of different styles of qigong that are taught and practiced for a variety of purposes. Spring Forest Qigong focuses on the use of qigong for healing.

"*Qi*" (pronounced chee) means energy, air or breath, vitality, or the Universal force of life. "*Gong*" means to work, use, practice, transform, cultivate or refine. Put simply, qigong means using this vital life energy to create a healthy mind and body. Through qigong we can heal not only physically, but emotionally, mentally and spiritually as well. In truth, this type of integrated healing is the only way we can be completely healed. Through the practice of qigong we can experience the perfect balance we are meant to have. Qigong combines meditation, focused concentration, breathing techniques and body movements to activate and cultivate our "vital energy" as it flows through the invisible energy channels, the meridians, of the body. Acupuncture is also based on the energy channels or meridians in the body.

Many people in the West first became familiar with acupuncture in the 1970's through newspaper columnist James Reston. During a trip to China, Reston had an emergency appendectomy and the doctors used acupuncture to ease his pain and promote faster healing. He was so impressed he wrote a column about his experience. Since that time interest in acupuncture has soared and millions of people in the West have made use of it.

Like western medicine acupuncture is very useful and can very effectively treat symptoms. Yet neither acupuncture nor western medicine treats the whole person or the underlying causes of the disease or pain. Also, you cannot treat yourself with acupuncture. Instead, you must turn that responsibility over to someone else. You have to go to see an acupuncturist just as you have to go to see a doctor.

Tens of millions of Chinese practice one style of qigong or another everyday. This ancient discipline is one of the most powerful self-healing practices ever developed by mankind. It is truly a wonder of our world and many people consider the results of qigong to be miraculous. In fact, qigong is one of the corner stones of traditional Chinese medicine.

In the past few decades, China has conducted numerous studies of qigong. These studies have shown that qigong can effectively help people in the prevention and healing of many diseases. Still, even in China, much of qigong teaching remains esoteric or hidden in mysterious secrets. Many qigong masters only reveal limited information to their students forcing the student to rely on the master instead of becoming the master of his or her own body and life. Most qigong masters teach that it takes years, decades or even an entire lifetime to learn how to use the universal energy to help others to heal. That is the way their masters taught them.

While there are many qigong techniques and movements that are difficult to learn and do take years of study and practice, it is not necessary to spend years to learn how to use qigong to help heal your body, have abundant energy and feel better. Qigong can be very simple to learn. You can learn Spring Forest Qigong very quickly and experience its powerful healing benefits from the very beginning.

How Qigong Works - The Essence of Qigong

If everything is a form of energy, then what is energy? Just like Tao, the law or principle of the universe in Chinese philosophy, energy cannot be explained. Therefore, something that can be explained is not energy. Energy cannot be created or destroyed. But what is the original form of this energy?

Let me share with you a conversation between my young son and me. One evening I saw my son sitting on the floor gazing at the sky. It was nine o'clock. I came to him and said,

"Ming, it's time for bed now." He woke up from his dreaming and said to me, "Daddy, may I ask you a question?"
"Yes, of course." I replied.

"What kind of thing was I before I was born?"

"You were a tiny baby in mother's womb."

"Then what was I before that?"

"Mother and father loved each other and one day we decided to have you. That was how you came into being."

"Then what was I before that?"

"You silly boy. It's time to go to bed. When you grow up you will know."

I reached out my arms and held him up and tried to carry him to bed.

"But what happens after I grow up?"

"You will be as big as father and then you will go to college and

11

then you will have your children." I tried to make the conversation short.

"Then I will grow old."

"Yes, that's for sure."

"Then I will be as old as great grandma."

"Yes, you are right."

"Then I will die."

"Yes, everybody will die." Of course, my son did not actually understand the concept of death. He had heard about death from his great grandma who was eighty-five years old and had babysat him since he was born. Almost everyday when she fed him, she would say "Ming, you have to eat and eat more so that you can grow faster. Great grandma will not live long and I might die next year. But I want to see you go to school, and then college, and then...." So my son adopted the word "death" from his great grandma.

Then, he asked, "What's after that?"

I looked at the sky and thought I found a very smart answer for him, "You will change into a star in the sky, like that most bright one over there." I pointed to the sky while I was talking.

He looked at the sky, paused a while, and then said, "What's after that?"

Looking at him, I could not say any thing and at last I said, "You really need to go to bed now."

As an adult, when we hear a conversation like this we might

say, "Hey, kids are so full of imagination. They ask the darndest questions." Yet when we sit down and really think about what they are asking, we can feel puzzled ourselves. Yes. What was before that? What was at the very beginning? Where are we from and where will we return? And what will happen after that?

Those simple questions are not so simple to answer and as ordinary beings we might stop asking or finally give up, yet ancient Chinese masters did not give up.

The ancient Chinese researchers studying this universal energy stayed with these simple questions and through their lifetimes of study and research, eventually uncovered the mystery. These Taoist masters discovered that *everything comes from the emptiness and returns to the emptiness.*

In the very beginning, the whole universe was in the state of emptiness. When this emptiness came to a breaking point, two kinds of energy were formed—Yin energy and Yang energy.

Those two kinds of energy or *Qi*, form everything in the universe including matter. We, too, are formed by these two kinds of *Qi*—Yin and Yang. Yin represents something feminine, passive, and spiritual; Yang represents something masculine, active, and physical. Examples of Yin would be woman, water, spiri¬tual life, and earth. Examples of Yang would be man, fire, the physical body, and sky.

Yin and Yang energies attract each other and need each other to exist, yet they must be in a good balance. Either too much Yin or too much Yang will cause an imbalance. These imbalances form blockages in the body. Colds, arthritis, depression, tumors, etc, are simply the symptoms of the imbalance of Yin and Yang. These blockages keep energy from flowing freely throughout the energy channels of the body.

We have many energy channels in our body. There are twelve main channels plus eight reservoir channels and each channel has a specific purpose. The main channels carry energy to wherever energy is needed in the body and extra energy in the main channels flows into the reservoir channels where the body draws on energy when the main channels run low. Blockages in the main channels and reservoir channels prevent energy from getting to parts of the body that need energy causing body functioning to slow down or stop and we feel sick.

Imagine these energy channels are like a river. When the river is flowing smoothly everything is fine. Farmers can take water from the river for their crops. Cities can use water from the river for people to drink. You can even have fun floating on an inner tube down the river on a hot day. But if something happens to cause a blockage in the river many problems can occur. Downstream the river can dry up and there will be no water to drink or for the farmer's crops, while upstream the river can overflow its banks and cause flooding.

With a river it's easy to see that a blockage can cause a lot of problems. It is the same with the energy channels in our bodies. If we want to get well and to feel our best we have to keep these energy channels open so the energy flows smoothly and freely. When we have blockages we need to open or remove these blockages and rebalance the Yin-Yang energy in our bodies.

This is where qigong can help. Through qigong practice we remove blockages so that energy can flow through the body in perfect balance. This balance brings healing, peak performance, inner peace, harmony and happiness.

Qigong exercise and meditation is an active and preventative way to heal the body, while medicine is a passive way to heal the body. Both play an important role, but qigong can potentially heal the body more effectively and possibly with perfection.

Of course, there are many wonderful things that modern medicine can do and I would never recommend that anyone stop seeing their doctor or stop following their doctor's advice. Instead, I believe that qigong can work very effectively with modern medicine as a complimentary practice.

A perfect healing heals the body physically, mentally, and spiritually at the same time. Qigong opens the door for holistic, perfect healing. This is needed more today than ever in the history of mankind. With the revolution of modern technology and computers, more and more people are working in their homes or in an office. Since much less physical work is required many more people develop Yin-Yang imbalances in the body.

As we have already discussed, Yin energy is something passive, while Yang energy is active. Thus, mental work belongs to Yin energy and physical work belongs to Yang energy. Since we tend to use more mental energy and have greatly cut down physical activities many of us have created an imbalance in both our physical and mental body. In order to heal we need to correct this imbalance and qigong is an ideal practice to help us achieve this goal.

More and more people in the world, including doctors, scientists, psychologists, nurses and other professionals are turning to qigong not only because of its simplicity and effective healing power but because they see a great need. Western medicine can be very effective and has helped hundreds of millions of people from suffering, but it has weak points:

- It is not a preventative medicine.
- It deals primarily with symptoms, not the cause.
- It focuses on the physical body only, ignoring the energetic levels of human beings, including the mental and spiritual dimensions.

- It can have side effects that potentially create more problems.
- It puts the patient in a passive role in the healing process.
- It is very costly.

Qigong addresses many of these weaknesses because qigong focuses on the cause of sickness and heals the body energetically by working physically, spiritually, and mentally. It can often heal the body faster and more completely with little or no side effects, a much lower cost, and the active healing involvement of the patient. At the same time, qigong can help prevent future problems.

What is Spring Forest Qigong?

Spring Forest Qigong (SFQ) is an advanced, simple and powerful form of qigong. I first introduced this unique form to people in 1994.

SFQ puts the power back in our hands. SFQ was created to help everyone realize that are we are born with the natural ability to heal ourselves, to detect energy blockages in the body, and to use our Qi to help others to heal themselves.

After being completely healed of pain myself, resulting from an injury and the depression that went along with it, I knew that there was something special in qigong and I searched for ways to share and help others. Qigong healing techniques have traditionally been very complex, difficult and cloaked in mystery. Through many years of research and practice, I have revised and simplified qigong movements and principles so they are easy to learn and fit into our daily lives.

Spring Forest Qigong makes the healing power of qigong simple, powerful and accessible to all of us.

Rewards and Benefits of Spring Forest Qigong

Learning and practicing Spring Forest Qigong brings many rewards. With enjoyable, easy to learn meditations and exercises that train the mind, breath, and posture, SFQ empowers you to:

- discover your natural ability to heal yourself
- acquire the power to help protect yourself from ill health; mentally, physically and spiritually
- learn knowledge and skills to continually strengthen your health, well-being, and mental outlook throughout your lifetime
- develop your natural capability for helping others to heal

Through practicing Spring Forest Qigong you put the power back in your own hands.

Health Benefits of Spring Forest Qigong

Spring Forest Qigong is an integrated form of healing, helping us to heal on all levels- physically, mentally/emotionally and spiritually. Although each person and situation is unique the benefits of practicing SFQ can include:

- Pain-free movement and greater flexibility
- A sense of contentment and peace
- Reduced stress and tension
- Improved metabolism, digestion, and elimination
- Balanced energy
- A more youthful appearance
- Increased awareness and mental acuity
- Increased strength and vitality

- Restore organs to their healthy, optimal functioning by giving them an "inner massage" and thus slowing the aging process

Healing Experiences with Spring Forest Qigong

The results experienced by my Spring Forest Qigong students have shown that practicing SFQ has helped in healing many sicknesses including:

- General pain: neck, shoulder, knee, back, arthritis, joint pain and postoperative pain.
- Migraine headaches, sinus problems & allergies
- Spinal problems
- Weight loss
- Hearing and vision problems
- Female and male organ problems
- Kidney and liver dysfunction
- Glandular dysfunction such as thyroid problems
- Diabetes problems
- Gallbladder and kidney stones
- Heart disease: heart attacks, congestive heart failure, recovery from heart surgery and general heart dysfunction
- Circulation problems
- Strokes
- Cancers
- Mental disorders: post-traumatic stress disorder, panic attacks, addictions, obsessive/compulsive disorder, hyperactivity, dyslexia
- Stress, anxiety, and depression
- Lung problems

- Autoimmune dysfunction such as AIDS & Lupus
- Bone marrow problems
- Comas
- Digestion problems

All of these wonderful benefits and results are possible because Spring Forest Qigong does not focus on symptoms. We focus on the root cause of all physical or mental illnesses -- the energy blockages in the body. By removing the blockages and restoring the natural energy balance in the body all of these results are possible and more.

The Question of Religion and Qigong

There are some people who ask whether qigong is a type of religion. I want to make it very clear that qigong is not a religion and has nothing to do with religion. Some might call qigong a philosophy but it is really a science. In fact, some Chinese masters refer to qigong as the "Body Science."

When people ask me if you have to be a certain religion to benefit from practicing Spring Forest Qigong, the answer is absolutely not. Whether you are Christian, Muslim, Jewish, Taoist, Hindu or Buddhist you can practice and experience the full benefits of qigong. You can practice any religion or none at all. It does not matter. I want to make this very clear.

The great Indian man of peace, Mahatma Gandhi, was once asked what religion he practiced. He answered by saying, "I am a Christian. I am a Muslim. I am a Hindu. I am a Jew." His message was clear. He believed that all people are brothers, that all women and men are equal and the same in the eyes of God. I believe that also, but that is my personal belief and has nothing to do with qigong.

Many years ago in China, I was in qigong training and was meditating deep inside a cave. This meditation lasted for several weeks. During the meditation I saw myself walk up to three men who were seated around a table talking together. As I got closer I recognized all three. The men were Jesus Christ, Buddha and Lao Tzu. The message to me was very clear: They were brothers.

Sometime later I was in a bookstore and my attention was drawn to a table. On the table were some books about Taoism, Buddhism, Christianity and Islam. I bought the books and read them. The spiritual message I got from each of the books was the same. The message is one of peace, love and forgiveness.

Whether you are a religious person or not is not an issue in Spring Forest Qigong. However, you must have love, kindness and forgiveness in your heart to experience the full power, the true joy and miracle of qigong. This I know to be true.

Awakening Your Natural Healing Ability

To be healed completely and perfectly we must remove the blockage or blockages in the body, balance the energy and keep it flowing smoothly. Most healing techniques, including modern medicine, deal only with the symptoms and not the root cause. These treatments can be very helpful but as long as the blockage remains and the energy is not flowing smoothly the pain or sickness will come back. Perhaps in the same way or perhaps with different symptoms, but the pain will return. Practicing qigong is a wonderfully effective way to remove energy blockages which are the root causes of pain and sickness.

In the past most qigong exercises were complicated and time consuming, making it difficult for the average person to learn and practice and even today many qigong masters do not explain the meaning or importance of the movements. Instead, they surround themselves and the ancient concepts they teach in mystery and then tell their students that it may take years to learn the exercises and experience the benefits. Even though qigong has been traditionally taught in this way for thousands of years I have found that it is unnecessary.

My personal experience and over twenty five years of qigong study with many wonderful masters has revealed to me that it is actually very simple to learn how to awaken your natural healing ability through qigong. That is why I created Spring Forest Qigong. In fact – you can start right now!

Helping Others Heal

You can use Qi (energy) to heal yourself. You can also use Qi to help others, because the principles are the same.

You will find it easy and simple to send energy out to help others heal.

A long time ago I asked different qigong masters how long it would take to learn to help heal others. Some said ten years; some said fifteen years; some even said fifty years.

However, I have learned it takes only two minutes! Follow my instructions and see for yourself.

- First hold your fingers in a position we call *swordfingers*. The tips of the little and ring fingers touch the first part of the thumb, forming a circle. The middle and index fingers rest together and point straight out.

- Point your *swordfingers* towards an area where your friend feels pain or discomfort (you will learn how to detect blockages in Level Two).

- Move your *swordfingers* around to break up the energy blockages.

- Open your fingers. Visualize energy shooting out from your fingers – you can use both hands or one. Energy goes into the part of the body where it has blockages whether pain, a stone, a tumor, or whatever.

- Visualize the energy changing blockages into air or smoke. Take hold of the air or smoke. Move it out of the body, and throw it to the earth. This energy blockage is extra energy in the body that you return to the universe. Keep pulling the air out until you feel the blockage is clear.

- While you are pulling out the blockage, repeat in your mind, "Blockages open. Pain is gone. You are completely healed." Say that loudly with great confidence in your mind.

- Use your palm(s) to give healing energy back to the area where you removed the blockage by moving your hand in and out nine times. Wear a smile on your face and move your hand(s) gently, because the energy will be more comforting.

Special notes:

1) Do not point *swordfingers* to the front of the heart, because the frequency of the energy does not agree with the hearts energy. This will not harm the heart, but it is not helpful.

2) Do not pull energy from the front of the heart or the top of the head, because that is not helpful. (This is discussed in considerable detail in Level Two.)

In Spring Forest healing, the more energy you send out to heal others, the more you will receive.

The keys are:

- Always call upon your master's energy to tap a tremendous resource. When your master's energy joins your energy, you will have much more energy to use.

- While you are doing the healing, visualize universal energy coming into your body through every cell and gathering in your lower dantian. In this way, you replenish the energy you are sending out.

- When you are finished ask your friend to take three deep breaths, rub his hands, and massage his face. These movements help him come out of the meditation without feeling spacey.

- Then say, "You feel better now!" or something encouraging like that instead of something such as, "Do you still feel the pain?" Because asking if they feel the pain could cause your friend to search for the pain and bring it back.

- You can also use sword fingers to help heal yourself.

- To make your healing more effective, have faith. Trust the universal/spiritual energy.

- Feel confident. Focus on how much you love people not

on success or failure. Embrace your eagerness to help friends. Focus on the honorable opportunity you have as you help yourself grow.

- Visualize the sickness, pain and discomfort as smoke. Or be creative and come up with another visualization to focus the power of your mind. *The stronger your focus and visualization the more successful your healing.*

Now that you have practiced your first healing technique, let's explore the four components of Spring Forest Qigong exercises and meditations.

Four Elements of Spring Forest Qigong

There are four elements to each Spring Forest Qigong exercise: Mind and Visualization, Breath, Postures and Body Movements and Sound. Learning about these components and being aware of them when practicing Spring Forest Qigong will enhance the benefits.

The Mind/Visualization

The first element of SFQ exercises is the mind and visualization.

In order to demonstrate the power of our mind let's try a game called "The Finger Growing Game." This game helps us experience how energy follows intention and illustrates the power of our minds.

The Finger Growing Game

To begin find the lines at the bottom of your hands where your wrists begin. Put these two lines together then put your palms together. Compare the length of your fingers. Most people have fingers that are slightly longer on one hand.

Next, raise the hand with the shorter fingers above your head and rest the hand with the longer fingers on your lower stomach. Slightly stretch open the hand that is above your head. Put a smile on your face, close your eyes and repeat this message in your mind, "My fingers are grow¬ing longer, longer, longer... They are growing longer, longer, longer and still longer. Say it to yourself with complete confidence. Simply know that your fingers are growing longer. Continue for about a minute then open your eyes and read on.

Minute up? Okay, compare your hands again. Your shorter fingers became longer, didn't they! (If they didn't don't worry…)

Now, open your hands. Say in your mind, "my fingers are back to normal." You only need to say it once. Line your palms up at the wrists again and compare your fingers now and see what's happened. They should be back to the same length they were when you started.

Want to play some more? Put the hand with the longer fingers up in the air and place your other hand on your stomach. This time we want the longer fingers to become shorter. Please slightly open the hand with longer fingers and say in your mind, "My fingers are becoming shorter, shorter, shorter, shorter...." Focus your mind on the fingers and feel the energy flowing in the fingers. Say in your mind, "My fingers are becoming shorter, shorter, shorter. My fingers are becoming shorter, shorter, and even shorter." Again, do this for 30 seconds to a minute.

Find the lines at the end of your palms, put them together and compare your fingers now. Did the longer fingers become shorter? We don't want to leave them that way, so open your hands and say in your mind, "my fingers go back to normal." Compare your fingers now.

Isn't this amazing? Congratulations! You've just experienced the power of Qi and using your mind to direct that powerful energy.

Our brain is very powerful, yet we only use a very small portion of it, between two and ten percent. If we could apply an additional one or two percent of our brain to the health of our bodies think of what miracles would happen in our lives!

When we repeated that our fingers were growing longer or becoming shorter, we focused our mind in our fingers and the fingers either grew longer or became shorter according to our message. Why does this work? This game works because we simply put energy into our fingers causing finger joints to open or close thus causing the fingers to become longer or shorter. Do you see a hint here for healing yourself?

We get sick because our channels are not completely open. When energy cannot flow easily to reach the organs that need the energy, part of the functioning of these organs has to shut down. That is why we feel sick.

Since we can use our mind to make our fingers grow in only a minute, we can easily use our mind to open up all the energy channels in our bodies. If you say in our mind "My pain is gone. I am completely healed." and repeat this message just like you did with your fingers you certainly can open those blocked channels in the same way. Once the channels open more energy flows to the organs that need energy causing the functions of the organs return to normal and the sickness to disappear. That is why some people experience an overnight "miracle." And once energy channels open, you only need to keep them open to maintain that quality of health.

I completely agree with the saying "the body cannot make the mind sick, but the mind can make the body sick." Our minds are very powerful. Much more powerful than our physical body. If we think in a positive way, positive things will happen. If we think in a negative way, negative things will happen. When you practice qigong and in your daily life, please consider the importance of your mind.

Good, Better, Best

One way to practice directing our minds positively is to follow the principle of "good, better, best." In Spring Forest Qigong there is no right or wrong, only good, better, best. Each movement has been designed to enhance the flow of energy in your body and bring it into balance. There is no such thing as bad or negative energy. Energy is energy. It only causes problems in the body, mind or emotions when the energy is not in balance or is in the wrong place.

Some people become so focused on trying to do the movements "perfectly" they do not allow themselves to relax completely. All of the movements of Spring Forest Qigong are designed to help you remove energy blockages in the body in multiple ways so there is no need for you to be concerned about getting it "right." If your hands are not in the "perfect" position, if you do not have full range of motion, do not be concerned. Simply allow your body and mind to fully relax as you move through the movements.

When you learn and practice in the best way you can you are always helping to balance the energy in the body and that will always be good. Please don't miss out on the good benefit you will receive by striving to be "perfect." Good is wonderful and as you continue to practice you will naturally get better and better and the benefits you receive will continue to grow.

The Password

Another helpful way to direct our minds is the Spring Forest Qigong password: "I am in the universe. The Universe is in my body. The universe and I combine together as one." The password is a powerful intention, aligning us with the energy of the universe.

Before you practice Spring Forest Qigong exercises or meditation silently repeat in your mind this password:

I am in the universe.

The universe is in my body.

The universe and I combine together.

The password connects us with the universal energy.

If you are a religious or spiritual person when you say the password you may wish to say it in a somewhat different way. In order to make it more meaningful for you personally, you may wish to use words that have deep meaning for you in your religious tradition. For instance when you refer to the universe you may wish to use a different word such as: God, Jesus, Allah, Great Spirit or Buddha. This is beautiful. As long as the words you choose represent love, kindness, forgiveness and a limitless source of healing power they will be helpful in bringing you to a place of peace and wonderful healing energy. It is not the specific words that matter, but rather, the meaning behind them.

We are all part of the universal energy. Once we open ourselves up to the universe, the universal energy is with us and gives our body whatever kind of energy it needs and automatically returns to the universe what it does not need.

Remember, everything comes from the emptiness and returns to the emptiness. Everything is energy in different forms and there is not really good energy or bad energy until we think of it as good or bad or put it in the wrong position. It is helpful to remember that sickness is only misplaced or extra energy in the body and that we can heal simply by returning the extra energy back to the universe.

Once we say the password: "I am in the universe. The universe is in my body. The universe and I combine together." We draw on the universal energy to balance the energy in our body.

Give it a try! Begin training your mind. Practice the first 3 Spring Forest Qigong exercises:
   Beginning of the Universe,
   Forming of the Yin and Yang and
   Moving of Yin and Yang.
These fundamental SFQ exercises are described on page 78, 80 & 82.

Breathing

The second element of SFQ exercises is the breath.

Breathing is the most important element of SFQ. Slow, deep and controlled breathing has long been a vital element of all forms of Qigong. Medical science has found that people with fewer breaths per minute are on the whole healthier than those who breathe more rapidly.

One of the most important systems in our bodies is the nervous system, which controls the messages and information traveling in the body. Blockages in the nervous system prevent messages from being delivered, creating problems.

The nervous system consists of two parts: the parasympathetic nervous system and the sympathetic nervous system. When we inhale energy goes to the sympathetic nervous system and when we exhale energy reaches the parasympathetic nervous system. When we take longer breaths we send more energy to both nervous systems, which is why people who practice tai chi, qigong, yoga, or meditation usually enjoy a long healthy life and why people with chronic sicknesses often find relief through deep, gentle breaths.

It is often said that one dog year is equal to seven human years. A dog breathes twenty-seven times a minute and usually lives between ten and fifteen years. On the other hand, a tortoise breathes two to three times a minute and we can easily find a tortoise over one hundred years old. An average human being breathes seventeen times a minute. Through qigong and meditation, we slow down the rhythm of our breathing, which can help us to live longer, like the slow breathing tortoise.

In Spring Forest Qigong, we practice "Energy Breathing."

Step One: Breathing through your Skin

As you inhale, concentrate your mind in your skin and visualize the universal, unconditional love energy coming into your body through every cell and collecting in the lower dantian, which is deep behind the navel. As you exhale visualize any sickness or extra energy that is no longer needed shooting out from every cell of the body and returning to the end of the universe.

Once you are comfortable "breathing through your skin" add the next step, "joining the Qi."

Step Two: Joining the Qi (Energy)

As you inhale, draw your navel in a little. As you exhale, loosen your lower stomach and let it out a little. Do this gently, remembering that there is no need to force the breath and that it is not helpful to struggle. Simply relax and let the breath flow as effortlessly as possible.

Gently directing the breath in this way through "energy breathing" will allow the yin and yang energy in the body to join together. The upper part of the body, starting from the bellybutton, belongs to yang energy, male energy. The lower part of the body belongs to yin energy, female energy. When the body gets sick, one of the reasons is the yin and yang energy is out of balance and not communicating properly. Energy coming in through inhaling is yin and energy given out through exhaling is yang. Through energy breathing when we inhale we hold yin energy in the upper part of the body and when we exhale we guide yang energy into the lower stomach. This allows the yin and yang energy to communicate and join together.

My very good friend and student, Patrick, is a psychologist searched for many years to find additional methods to help his patients. Patrick has found that through this simple, relaxed way of breathing people experience enormous positive changes in their mental health.

Energy Breathing feels good and is great for your health!

Give it a try! Practice Energy Breathing along with 2 SFQ active exercises:
Breathing of the Universe and
Joining of Yin and Yang.
These SFQ exercises are described on pages: 84 and 86.

Postures and Body Movements

The third element of SFQ exercises is posture and movement.

Postures and movements are important when practicing Qigong because they help open the energy channels in the body. Simply opening the hands, for example, opens six main channels that begin in the hands. These include lung and large intestines channels, which begin in the thumb and the index finger, and heart channels, which begin in the middle and little fingers.

Some postures can give immediate and noticeable benefit: when you have a headache, cough, or stuffy nose, hold both hands above your head for five minutes and you will find that the cough or other symptom gradually stops. When you have a bloody nose in your right nostril, raise your left hand above the head for a minute and you will find that the blood stops without having to stick tissue paper into the nose. Those techniques work because raising your hands opens the lung channels, heart channels, and stomach channels, many of which run through the nose area. Replenish energy in these channels and symptoms disappear.

Spring Forest Qigong is very good for opening channels in the body largely because of its wonderful movements and postures. Different postures and movements open different channels and create different directions for the energy to flow.

When our energy channels are open, they send energy to every part of the body, keeping the body and mind in good shape. When the energy is flowing smoothly through our body's energy channels we feel good; physically, mentally, emotionally, spiritually. However, when our energy channels are blocked we feel sick. The blockages may result in physical or mental problems, or both. This, of course, raises the question, what causes the energy channels to become blocked?

What Causes Energy Blockages

There are six main causes of energy blockages:

1. Unbalanced Emotion
2. Nutrition
3. Weather and Seasons
4. Environment
5. Wrong medication
6. Injury

UNBALANCED EMOTION

First, let's talk about emotion. Unbalanced emotion is the biggest cause of blockages in the body. Too much or too little of any emotion can create blockages.

In general, Chinese medicine tells us that overexcitement and excessive happiness causes damage to the heart energy. Anger and anxiety damage the liver energy. Fear damages the kidney energy. Sadness and depression damage the lung energy. Too much thinking damages the energy of the stomach and pancreas system.

Our ancient wisdom asks us to stay calm in order to keep the Yin and Yang energy in a good balance. When the Yin energy and Yang energy are not in a good balance, the body is affected and may even be in trouble.

How can even too much of a "good" emotion cause damage? Let's look at how over-happiness can cause damage to the heart. When a person is very excited, the energy heats the heart first. Excess energy then travels up to the brain and once the energy gets into the brain it can become stuck, because the channel between the torso and the head is very narrow. Just like an over-filled balloon can explode, this excess energy can result in a stroke or heart attack. Many times I have received calls from people to cancel an appointment at the last minute because their grandma or grandpa or another elderly person had a heart attack or stroke at a wedding party, surprise party, etc.

How can too much anger create damage? Anger causes energy to collect in the liver. If this energy is too much and not removed from the liver soon enough, a blockage gradually forms and our liver becomes sick. The names of different diseases and illnesses created by the blockage differ, but they are the symptoms, while the energy blockage is the root of the sickness.

Please don't misunderstand. Emotions are good things; using them appropriately is the key. Even though emotions can cause blockages in the body, emotions can also help remove blockages when we use them properly. Here is an ancient Chinese story.

The governor of a county had been sick for a long time. He seldom talked and felt depressed all the time. He had no appetite even for delicious food. He had been to many good doctors, but nothing changed. Instead, he was getting worse.

One day a famous doctor came to the town and the governor sent his family to invite the doctor to the house to see him. The doctor came. After listening to his stories, the doctor packed up all his tools and prepared to leave. He said, "You are just doing fine except your menstruation is abnormal. That is all."

When the governor heard this he could not believe his ears. In China, if you say a man has menstruation, this is the biggest insult. When he really realized what the doctor said, he was so mad that he drove the doctor out of the house and almost killed him.

After that day, whenever he thought of this doctor's words, he felt so angry. He told people how terrible this doctor was, threw all his expensive medicine away and decided not to see doctors anymore. He loved to tell anyone who came to see him the story, his appetite gradually came back and his depression disappeared. He was healthy again.

A few months later, he met a friend who was a doctor. This friend was surprised to see how healthy he was and asked him how he got healed. He told his friend the whole story with laughter. His friend listened with great attention and when he finished his story, said to him, "No wonder he is a famous doctor. He used your emotions to heal you. He used your anger and laughter to heal your depression – without medicine!"

This story makes a good point about using emotion constructively. It also makes a strong point about the power of the mind, doesn't it?

Anger, fear, resentment, anxiety, doubt, even too much excitement can all cause blockages in our energy channels. These blockages can lead to one type of illness or another, but the illness is only the symptom, not the cause.

What the famous doctor did was help the governor to restore balance in his mind and body. This is exactly what Spring Forest Qigong does. Spring Forest Qigong teaches you how to restore balance in a natural and easy way.

Let me share a couple of Spring Forest Qigong stories. The first illustrates how in the process of restoring balance Spring Forest Qigong can not only provide dramatic physical benefits but emotional, mental and spiritual benefits as well.

When I first came to the United States as an exchange teacher back in 1992, I met a woman named Esther who has since become my very good friend.

Many years before, Esther was stricken with a very rare lung disease. She had to be on oxygen 24 hours a day and couldn't go anywhere without wheeling her oxygen canister along with her. The doctors told her she needed a lung transplant or she would be on oxygen for the rest of her life.

Esther's son had heard wonderful stories about how people had experienced miraculous health benefits from Qigong. He heard about a class I was teaching at a local high school and asked his mother to come. Even with his encouragement, Esther did not want to come to my class. She was a very religious person and was afraid her church wouldn't approve. Esther says her son "dragged me kicking and screaming" to that first class.

The class was one night a week for eight weeks. On week seven, Esther, her husband and son walked into my class all smiling. Esther was walking without oxygen. It was the first time in more than a decade that she could breathe without oxygen let alone walk without it. She was so happy.

Esther has shared her story many times. She never expected that anything good would come from going to my class and was totally surprised that her body had been healed. But what was even more amazing to her was the emotional change that had taken place. Even before her illness, Esther says she was always "one crabby S.O.B." but not anymore.

Esther learned how to balance her energy and she experienced a perfect healing. She was healed not only physically, but mentally, emotionally and spiritually.

The next Spring Forest Qigong story relates to using SFQ to help relieve stress. Doctors know that stress is one of the biggest causes of disease; not only physical illness but also mental and emotional problems. In fact, stress may be the biggest threat to a person's physical, mental and emotional health and well being.

Stress can cause anxiety, anger, fear and other emotions that cause energy blockages in the body. Left unbalanced, these energy blockages often result in one form of illness or another. That is why many doctors recommend that their patients find ways to relieve stress.

By themselves, the breathing and movement in Spring Forest Qigong are excellent ways to relieve stress. When you add visualization and the healing sounds, SFQ becomes an even more powerful method of stress reduction. In fact, when you regularly practice Spring Forest Qigong you may find that day to day stresses don't seem so bad anymore.

Practicing SFQ keeps your energy more balanced and helps shift your perception of yourself and the world. When stressful situations occur, they are not as likely to be heavy burdens that weigh you down or keep you from performing your best. You can feel happy where you are right now, knowing that life is for happiness, and as with all things, this too shall pass.

A few years ago a young woman in her early twenties came to see me. She was married with young children. When her doctor found lumps in her breasts she had surgery but the lumps returned. She had a second surgery and the lumps returned again, even larger than before.

When she came to see me it was obvious that her problems were caused by stress. She worried about so many things. Material things. Financial things. Would there be enough money? Would her children get the right education? So much worry. So much stress. I recommended that she take things easy. Whatever happens, happens. Whatever doesn't happen, doesn't happen. Don't focus too much on material things or get caught up in worries. Instead, focus on how wonderful life is. Life is short. You don't have time to worry about all these things. Focus on positive things.

Then I used the techniques of Spring Forest Qigong to help her in removing the blockages in her body and to help her to balance her energy. After her first visit her tumor was 95 percent gone. It was down to the size of a pea. After her second visit it disappeared completely.

Later, she wrote me a letter. She said that after her first visit she felt so wonderful. She said that she noticed all the beautiful things that were all around her and that for the first time in her life she really noticed the birds singing and how wonderful they sounded. She noticed that the grass was green and had never realized that grass was green before!

Of course, she had heard birds and looked at the green grass before, but her experience of those things had changed. She had experienced beauty and gratitude in a deeper way. So many people go through life not noticing all the beautiful things the world has to offer. A smile. A laugh. A sunset. Or, that the grass is green.

There is nothing wrong with material things. There is nothing wrong in wanting a beautiful house or a fine car or wanting the best things in life for your children. All of these things are fine. Yet focusing too much on them, struggling to get them, fearing that you won't have them, all of this causes your energy to be out of balance. This leads to stress and negative emotions that cause blockages which can result in disease. And, what is disease but dis-ease.

Try not to focus on material things at the expense of spiritual things. It's not worth the price you will pay. Instead, try to keep all things in their proper balance. Life is for happiness. By practicing Spring Forest Qigong you help keep your energy balanced and bring that happiness into your life more and more each day. You may even find that things in your life begin to fall into a perfect balance quite naturally and beautifully.

NUTRITION

Nutrition is the second biggest factor that causes energy blockages in the body. Each day we eat two or three meals plus snacks. When we do not eat well our body's energy gets out of balance. As we have learned, everything is made up of energy (Qi). Naturally, the food we eat has energy that affects our bodies and different types of food have different qualities of energy.

Tips for Healthy eating:

- *Whenever possible, eat things locally produced.* Our bodies and nature are one. We live on the land with plants and plants grow well because of the harmony between their energy and the energy of the land. When we eat food produced locally, our body ingests the optimal energy (Qi) we need for the area in which we live.

- *Drink Yin-Yang water.* Yin-Yang water is Taoist medicine water. It helps balance the energy in the body. It is especially good for the digestive system and can also help with diarrhea or constipation. In the morning I drink a glass of Yin-Yang water with honey. I make Yin-Yang water in this way. I take half a glass of spring water and half a glass of boiled water and mix them together. Then I put one or two spoonfuls of honey into the water and drink it while it is still warm. (Don't refrigerate or put ice into it.) Yin-Yang water plus honey is very good cleansing water. (Of course, you need to consult your doctor before you give this water to babies and young children. It is rare but some people are allergic to honey.)

- *Eat honey.* Honey is considered a wonderful medicine in China. Bees have to visit millions of flowers before they can produce a pound of honey. This makes honey a powerful herbal medicine.

- *In the spring and summer avoid eating too much deep fried and spicy food.* This can easily cause spleen problems. Also, in general, spicy food is not helpful for the liver.

- *If you have stomach troubles avoid acidic food* because that can cause problems for the stomach.

- *If you need to be careful about your heart avoid sweet foods* and favor spicier foods instead.

- *Put healing energy into your food.* In China there is a famous saying, "Eat to Heal" and mealtime is considered the best time to help balance energy in the body.

Those are some general tips. However, you don't need to become an expert on nutrition or Chinese cooking to eat a healthy balance diet. And, by learning and practicing Spring Forest Qigong you will be removing blockages in your body and maintaining the energy balance you need to stay healthy.

WEATHER & SEASONS

Changes in the weather and the seasons can also cause blockages in our bodies. The earth rotates as it revolves around the sun to give us days, nights, and different seasons. When the weather or the seasons change the energy frequency of our body may not be in harmony with the energy frequency of the world around us. In other words, our internal energy may not have "caught up" with what's happening energetically externally. That's why we see:

- As spring comes, more people have liver problems.
- As summer comes, more people have heart problems.
- As fall comes, more people have lung problems.
- As winter comes, more people have kidney problems.

When we practice Spring Forest Qigong we naturally adjust our energy to the changes of the weather before a blockage occurs. So, SFQ is an ideal way to prepare for the changing weather and seasons. Let's look at some other tips that can also help us remain balanced during these changes.

Ancient Chinese wisdom encourages us to follow the principles of nature so that we can achieve our health and longevity. Adjusting our sleeping patterns to mirror the seasons is one way to do that. In the spring everything is growing day and night, so it is best to get up early and go to bed late. In the summer everything is developing rapidly in nature, so we should also go to bed late in the evening and get up early. In the fall, it is a harvesting time, so we should go to bed early and get up early. And in the winter, the energy of everything turns inward to store energy for the spring, so we should go to bed early and not get up until the sun comes up.

For many of us it is either very difficult or not practical to follow this kind of schedule. In that case, simply following our qigong practice will help us adjust to the changes of the seasons so that we can balance the energy in the body before any major blockages occur to trouble us.

Besides the seasonal changes, other changes in the weather can cause energy imbalances in our bodies. Think of the power of a thunderstorm for example. It comes with a dramatic change in atmospheric pressure. Oftentimes, you can feel this change of pressure in your body, in your joints or sinuses for example. You can feel the change in the air around you. The air is another form of energy and you are feeling the quality of the energy changing.

Try to avoid practicing your qigong outside when the weather is going through dramatic change or when it is very windy outdoors. The changing quality of the energy in the air is very powerful and could interfere with your ability to balance your own energy. If this situation exists, try to practice indoors.

Some people say they can predict changes in the weather by the feelings they get in their joints or at the point of an old injury or broken bone. Again, their bodies are reacting to the changing energy in the atmosphere. In a more subtle example, too many cloudy or rainy days in a row can cause people to feel lethargic or even depressed. Once again, it is a question of balance.

We may not be able to make the weather the way we want it on a given day, but by practicing Spring Forest Qigong we will be continuously maintaining the energy balance in our own bodies. In this way, we take our personal well being into our own hands.

ENVIRONMENT

Now we come to the environment, another factor that can create blockages in the body.

In western society when people discuss harmful effects of the environment, they often refer to different types of pollution: air pollution, water pollution, sound pollution, etc. These things certainly do impact us. For example, there are people who have developed such strong sensitivities to chemicals in the environment they become deathly ill. For some people who suffer from environmental illness, exposure to certain chemicals has so badly damaged their immune systems their bodies are unable to make use of their natural defense mechanisms.

Their bodies are now terribly out of balance. Western medicine often treats such cases by placing the patient in an environment free from any chemical exposure to give the immune system the opportunity to strengthen itself. These "clean rooms" are made only of glass, ceramics, or stainless steel.

I have worked with many people who have had chemical sensitivities and immune system dysfunction. By using the techniques of Spring Forest Qigong, I have seen wonderful recoveries in these people and seen them restored to perfect health.

Environmental pollution is one aspect of how the environment can cause energy blockages in the body. Another environmental factor relates to the Chinese art of Feng Shui. One of the factors that Feng Shui stresses is the importance of the location and direction of the home in which we live. Feng Shui is a study of Qi, energy from the earth, sun, and moon. Whether we are aware of it or not the energy from the earth, the sun and the moon influence our lives and when these energies are combined harmoniously they create a good, healthy place for living.

According to Feng Shui different parts of a building have different energy and each object has its own magnetic field and energy frequency that positively or adversely influences our body's energy. We can adjust for this by arranging furniture in an optimal location and direction so that the frequency of the energy from these objects meets the frequency of our body's energy. As an example, it is best not to place a mirror facing your bed, because the mirror's energy is too invasive and will affect your sleeping quality.

The following stories are two examples of how Feng Shui can impact the energy in our bodies.

The first example involves some friends who invited me to dinner and to see the "Feng Shui" of their house. I went outside to look around the street. Their front door was facing the south. I said you have a very good location for doing business. They told me that in the past two years, their business had developed ten times. But when I went down to the basement I told them that everyone in the house unfortunately had lower back problems, for women in the right side of the lower back, and for men on the left side.

They were very surprised that the design of the basement could cause physical problems in the body. They said before they moved into the house, they did not have any back pain problems, but now it was exactly as I said. In order to balance the energy in their basement, I asked them to find something to fill up one corner and then on the opposite wall put up a mirror facing that corner. They did it and their back problems went away.

The next example involves a couple who came to see me for depression and cancer. The husband had depression and lower back pain, and the wife had depression and breast cancer. She had breast cancer before and one breast had been removed. Now the cancer had spread to the other side and her doctor wanted to remove the other breast, but she did not want to do that. She wanted to find a new solution to her illness.

They attended one of my classes, and after practicing the SFQ exercises and a series of healing sessions they both recovered. They were very happy about that. At their last visit I asked them whether their children had depression. They said all their children were very beautiful kids, but none of them finished their high school education, and they were all involved in gangs and drugs and even tried to commit suicide.

My intuition told me that they had a big tree right in front of the entrance to their home that blocked the energy in the house and caused the depression of the family. They did have a large tree in front of their house but they could not understand how it could affect their family in that way. The oak tree was very healthy. How could a tree like that cause a blockage in the house and the people's bodies in the house?

I explained to them the important concept that energy is energy. *There is no good energy or bad energy.* However, energy can be too much, too little or misplaced. When we see an object our eyes capture the frequency of that object's energy and sends the information to the brain. When the brain receives the information, through the chemical activities in the body, the brain classifies all the information and gives an answer to the information. Each day when they opened or closed the door, the same type of energy frequency was captured by the eyes, which caused the same kind of chemical activities in the body. Gradually the same kind of energy would gather in the body, which would influence the thinking format. That is why the depression occurred. I told them either to move their house or put a big mirror in the house facing out to the tree in order to help balance the energy between the tree and the house.

Every object has its own frequency of energy. If we put it in the right place, the energy will be good for our body. If we put it in the wrong place, it will cause damage in our body. This may all be very new to you and sound very strange, so allow me to explain further.

You may remember from your high school science class that everything in the world, including every cell in your body, is made up of atoms. These atoms are constantly in motion and within them are even smaller, highly charged particles that are also constantly in motion. Within those particles are even smaller particles that are also constantly in motion, and so on. Motion and Energy. Again, everything is a type of energy. Scientists are still searching for ways to accurately measure the motion of the smallest of these particles.

For our purposes, the point is that everything is a type of energy and that energy vibrates at a certain rate creating its own magnetic field. Different magnetic fields react to others in different ways. Some attract. Some repel. It is how these different magnetic fields react to each other that makes all the difference.

If you want to live in a place with wonderful Feng Shui, look for a place where there are a lot of tall, healthy trees, and many birds and animals such as deer, foxes and geese. Why? Because growing trees reflect and enhance the energy (the Qi) in the land. Animals such as foxes, deer, and geese are very sensitive to that energy, so when you find a place with those qualities it is certainly a good place to build your house.

Having such a wonderful place to live is indeed very helpful for our body's energy system, but it is not necessary in order to be happy and healthy. Since qigong strengthens our body's magnetic field, we can change the energy of our house and environment simply by practicing Spring Forest Qigong. When your body's magnetic field is stronger than that of your house, nothing can affect your energy. Instead, your energy will affect everything and everyone around you. At home your family and pets will benefit from your energy. At work people will benefit from your energy as well. You may even find that difficult people are attracted to you and will not make trouble for you because they feel safe being with you and need your comforting, love energy.

This may take time but can even happen overnight. I have seen it happen time and time again. Balancing your own energy is very, very powerful and can have untold benefits for you and everyone around you.

WRONG MEDICATION

Another factor in creating energy blockages is wrong medication.

Modern medicine helps a great many people and modern medication can be a lifesaver. Yet, at the same time, there are problems. These problems are often related to wrong prescriptions, side effects and inaccurate diagnoses.

In 1995, a medical report on television said that in the previous ten years in the United States, the number of people who died of wrong medication was more than the number of people who died in the Vietnam War. In 1997, the Journal of the American Medical Association reported that 105,000 patients died in hospitals from incorrectly prescribed medication that was properly administered.

Years from now we may hear more of the same terrible statistics because wrong medication will continue to harm people.

Frankly, even the right medicine can cause problems. When we listen to ads for medication on television, they list the possible side effects and some of these side effects sound worse than the symptoms they are treating. Also, it often happens that the more medication a person takes, the more medication a person has to take, with one prescription counterbalancing the side effects of another, and so on. This greatly increases the chances of harmful side effects because it is impossible to be certain how different medicines will interact.

One of the many wonderful things about Spring Forest Qigong is that there are no harmful side effects.

INJURY

Physical injury also causes blockages in the body. This is because all injuries can block energy (Qi) including cuts, carpal tunnel syndrome, sprained ankles, torn muscles, broken arms, contusions, etc. Furthermore, an injury in one part of the body can lead to blockages in another part of the body. For example, an injury to your knee can cause a blockage in the back or ankle.

Injuries can also lead to negative emotions that create even more blockages. Therefore, it is very important that whenever we suffer an injury, we work to maintain the energy balance in our body.

Let me share a story that one of my students told me. My student was watching her son play a little league baseball game when she noticed another mother arrive, limping. This woman was very athletic and generally very positive and energetic, but not this day. When my student asked her what was wrong, she said that she had twisted her ankle while jogging and that she was really "bummed" because she was supposed to play in a very important tennis match that afternoon and was going to have to cancel it.

My student told her friend she could help. She told her a little about Spring Forest Qigong and when the woman asked what she needed to do my student told her to simply close her eyes, put a smile on her face, place her tongue against the roof of her mouth, and take three gentle, deep breaths through her nose. She then asked the woman to say once in her mind, "My pain is gone. I am completely healed." After that, she said, just relax and think of something really beautiful, something that makes you happy.

Her friend followed the instructions and my student used the simple techniques she learned in my classes to help her friend. First, she used her "swordfingers" to break up the blockages around the ankle. Next, using her hand and her visualization skills, she "pulled" the energy blockages out and sent healing energy into the ankle. Then, to balance and help the energy in her friend's body flow smoothly she sent energy to her friend's *lower dantian* (the energy center deep behind the navel.)

When she was finished she asked her friend to take three deep, relaxed breaths through her nose and slowly open her eyes. My student was smiling when her friend opened her eyes and said, "Feel better now."

Her friend moved her ankle around a little and then stood up and took a few steps. Her eyes got as big as saucers and she smiled a big smile and said, "I can't believe it. It doesn't hurt. It feels perfect!" She was very happy. Later that night she called and said she felt so good and so relaxed that she had played the best game of tennis she'd played in years.

My student just smiled.

That story is very simple and very beautiful. It shows how easy it is to use Spring Forest Qigong to help others. It also shows how quickly things can change and that when you are relaxed and your energy is balanced and flowing smoothly you can experience "being in the zone" or what coaches often call "peak performance."

To review, the six main causes of energy blockages are unbalanced emotion, improper nutrition, changes in the weather and seasons, the environment, wrong medication and injury. With so many opportunities to create energy blockages it is no wonder that the energy in our bodies can become out of balance or stuck. Throughout the day each of us moves in and out of balance to greater or lesser degrees. That is one of the reasons practicing Spring Forest Qigong is so valuable and important. And the SFQ active exercises are particularly helpful in removing blockages and restoring energy flow and balance because of the specific postures and movements of the body.

Give it a try! Feel your body and observe the affect of movement while you practice more SFQ active exercises:

> *Harmony of Universal Energy,*
> *Seven Steps of New Life*
> *Harvesting of the Qi*

These exercises are described on pages 87 , 91 & 93.

The Sound

The fourth element of SFQ exercises is sound.

Different sounds have different vibrations. The frequency of the vibration can help open the channels too. Chanting certain sounds can be a powerful type of healing. From ancient times to today, people all over the world have been using chanting to remove blockages and heal the body. Chinese Taoist people teach people five sounds to heal the internal organs and they work very well. In Spring Forest Qigong we practice two sounds: o-o-h-m and m-u-a-ah. These two sounds carry very powerful energy signals and we practice these two sounds when we do the Small Universe sitting meditation.

If you like, you can begin to experience the energy of these sounds now. Open your hands and repeat "o-o-h-m" and "m-u-a-ah" in a very low tone. You may feel a tingly sensation throughout your body.

Give it a try! Experience the powerful vibration of sound by practicing the Small Universe Meditation.
This sitting meditation is described on page 103.

Three Principles of Spring Forest Qigong

Go into the emptiness

The first principle for practicing SFQ is: Go into the emptiness.

Ancient Chinese wisdom is that everything in our world is from the emptiness and will go back to the emptiness. You might call this place the mind of God or the source of all creation. It does not matter what you call it. I use the word emptiness and this emptiness a state of pure energy where we are one with the universe.

There are countless different styles of qigong and all of them teach the basic idea of using consciousness to go into the emptiness where thoughts ultimately cease or greatly diminish and sensory connections to our bodies fade. When we meditate our bodies naturally direct us to the emptiness in which we totally renew ourselves.

Let me ask you a question. What is the first thing you want to do when you have a headache? Most of us lie down and take a nap, if we can, and after the nap, we feel much better. Our headache may even be completely gone.

In the evening, after a long day of work, we may feel tired, and so, after we get everything done for the day, what do we usually do? Of course, we go to bed.

When we sleep we feel so relaxed and peaceful, because when we sleep we bring our mind and body into the emptiness, where we naturally get rid of our fatigue and any energy imbalances we developed during the day. This sleep is actually a very basic form of meditation and it happens automatically to all of us. Most of our daily energy blockages are opened and solved in this way – through simply sleeping. The deeper we sleep, the deeper we go into the emptiness and the faster our body is healed, so sleeping is a type of Qigong.

For healing the body and mind or for helping others to heal we need to go into the emptiness. The deeper a person can go into the emptiness, the place of perfect peace and pure energy, the higher their spiritual healing ability will become. This is done through meditation.

In order to meditate, first quiet your mind by bringing your awareness to one point in the body. This point could be the lower dantian, which is the energy center deep behind the belly button. This point could also be your heart, an image of the sun or the moon, etc. As you continue to effortlessly focus on this one point you will gradually have the sensation of stillness. As you stay in the stillness you will have the experience of not seeing or feeling anything, even your own existence. You don't know who you are or where you are and your whole body totally merges together with the universe.

Of course, it requires much practice before you can remain in the emptiness, yet the longer you can stay there, the faster your channels will open and stay open, and the more power you will have to use your own qi. As you practice SFQ meditations and active exercises you will be naturally increasing your ability to remain in the emptiness.

Keep it simple

The second principle for practicing SFQ is: Keep it Simple.

Although many qigong exercises are unnecessarily complicated and cloaked with mystery, qigong in its fundamental form is very simple. For instance, it is very easy to open energy channels. When you open your fingers, all the energy channels in the hands open and when you move your heels up and down, you open all six energy channels in the feet. So, as you can see, it is not necessary to learn and practice complicated movements to open channels and release blockages.

When you practice Spring Forest Qigong you will discover that keeping it simple is not only as effective, but can be even more effective than complicated movements. In truth, the most powerful techniques are usually the simplest.

Use your Consciousness

The third principle for practicing SFQ is: Use your Consciousness.

Consciousness is not the same as your conscious mind. Your conscious mind is what you are using now as you read these words and focus on their meaning. Your consciousness is the infinite part of you. It is your direct connection to the "emptiness," the source of all creation. Within that source we find infinite wisdom, power, energy and all we could ever need.

Our consciousness is always at work, sending us energy and messages. Yet our consciousness does not speak loudly and forcefully the way our conscious mind often does. Instead, our consciousness sends messages in very gentle, subtle ways, and so, we must quiet our minds and relax your bodies in order to receive these messages.

Through our SFQ practice we can learn to use our conscious mind in ways that open us up to our consciousness. For instance, when practicing the active exercises, move as slowly as possible. Try not to move too fast because the more slowly we move our hands, the more we feel the flow of energy *(Qi)* in the body. As we learn to relax through the movements, we learn to relax our minds. Thus we learn to direct our conscious mind in ways that do not block access to consciousness.

Another way to direct our conscious mind is being mindful of how our thought patterns influence the flow of energy *(Qi.)* Positive thoughts, for example, encourage health and rapidly direct Qi in optimal ways. Negative thoughts, on the other hand, block energy and create sickness. As we practice qigong we come to realize that mental power is more powerful than physical power.

Many people complain a lot about their lives and their bodies and these negative thoughts create energy blockages. In my childhood and teenage years, I suffered great abuse and many physical injuries which led to many physical and emotional problems. Then, as a young man, I suffered a very serious injury to both of my knees. Because the damage and pain was so great I could not walk and because the pain was so constant and intense I hated my body. At the time I could not see that my injury and pain had a positive purpose, but it did. My body was acting as a guide, trying to send me a message which for many years I did not understand.

While I knew some qigong, in those years I did not understand the true message and power of qigong healing. It was through desperately searching for ways to heal my body that I truly opened myself to qigong. That search has changed my life in so many wonderful ways and allowed me to use qigong to help many thousands of people. Once I understood the message that the pain in my body and in my heart held for me and acted upon it, the result was the greatest happiness I have ever known – and freedom from pain, anger and sickness. Viewing your life and your body in a positive way will bring you wonderful experiences as well.

The Keys to Your Success

Many people say that it is very difficult to meditate because it is so hard to quiet the mind. Especially when people are sick, they can find it hard not to think about their pain, sickness, or symptoms, making it difficult to relax and quiet their minds. When they try to meditate and it doesn't seem to work for them right away, they may feel disappointed and be tempted to give up.

Actually, Spring Forest Qigong meditations are very simple. Following some simple guidelines, you will find it easy. You may even find relief from discomfort or other symptoms immediately after you do the meditation exercises.

There are six keys that will lead to success when practicing Spring Forest Qigong meditations:

Faith

Confidence

Calling upon your master's energy

Visualization

Focus

Consistency

Faith

Life can be divided into two parts: material life (including our physical body) and spiritual life. Ignoring one can make the other meaningless. Most sickness starts in our spiritual life and then manifests physically.

Trust your soul and the universal energy. Trust those pioneers who studied the universal energy. Life cannot go well without faith and trust. Your own mind and body is the number one factor in healing yourself. When we get sick, healers and doctors only help facilitate healing. No one can really help us to heal unless we want to be healed. Even Jesus said that he could only help those who wanted to be helped. He also said that everyone could do what he did. That is remarkable and that is true. Our ancient wisdom taught us this truth thousands of years ago and the only thing we need to do is follow the guidance of the ages, trust this universal energy, this spiritual energy, and believe in ourselves.

When we have faith, our soul takes charge of our life. We can hear and trust our inner voice to guide us through whatever we encounter. We feel peaceful and our spirits are high, because we have faith in our soul. When we are still, quiet and at peace, we will hear this inner voice and need only follow its guidance.

Faith can give you courage to walk your life. Faith can give you confidence to overcome difficulties that others cannot manage. And faith can give you comfort when you are down.

Faith is not the same as belief. For instance, you do not have to believe that practicing qigong will heal your pain or sickness. Many of my students were quite skeptical when they first came to experience Spring Forest Qigong. They did not believe it could work – at least not for them. Yet they had the faith to try it and they experienced wonderful success.

Confidence

A trait of the most successful people of the world is unstoppable confidence. The same holds true for the greatest healers. If you are experiencing an illness, you have the opportunity to express your confidence.

Here are some of those ways:

- Regard your sickness as your teacher and your friend. Ask yourself why you are getting sick. An illness often relates to how you have been conducting your life. Have you been following the principles of nature? Have you been eating well? Have you been doing exercises and practicing qigong regularly? Have you been a happy person with universal love, kindness and forgiveness in your heart in all situations?

- Take your sickness as a positive warning. Listen to your inner voice. Follow it to understand your life, and you will certainly live a happier, healthier life.

- Accept the truth that everybody has the ability to heal herself or himself and to help heal others. We are born with these abilities and gifts and as you use them your confidence will build and you will be a more powerful healer.

- Hold in your heart that some day, through your continuous practice and with the help of your master's energy, you will get well.

Blockages are not formed in a day. Some blockages have been in the body for a long time. It may take time for you to let go of them. They stay in your body for a while as a teacher, in order to teach you to get back on the right track of life. When you are totally on track, the sickness disappears.

When you are sick, say to yourself, "I'm going to practice these exercises every day. I am sure I will get well. If not today, it will happen tomorrow. If not tomorrow, it will be the day after tomorrow, or the next week, or next month. I will absolutely get well!"

Sometimes, when you practice qigong exercises and meditation your symptoms disappear, however sometimes they seem to come back. This can be discouraging but actually it is part of the process of healing. You are clearing the root of the old messages in the body from a very deep level. Please don't give up. Keep doing the meditations and exercises and one day you will find it a joy to be free from pain. This is true in all aspects of life. If you do not give up when you meet difficulty eventually you will succeed. However, if you give up you will never have the chance to enjoy the fruit of your work.

My good friend and student, Gary, had this experience. Because of numerous injuries, he suffered from severe pain in his lower back for many years. He took pain killers every day just to be able to function. Gary had been to see many doctors, specialists and therapists. Some of them had helped to ease his pain but it never went away and every six months or so he would have a severe episode and his back would completely lock up on him.

When he first learned of Spring Forest Qigong he started to practice the exercises but felt even more pain and not just in his back. Because of this severe pain he stopped practicing. He stopped and started several times, always with the same result. When he finally told me about his experience and asked me what he was doing wrong I told him that his blockages had been there for many years and would take time to go away. I told him the pain was actually a very positive thing, because the pain was from the blockages breaking up, and that if he would just stay with the exercises he would have a wonderful result.

He took my advice, kept practicing and within a week he woke up one morning and all the pain in his back was gone – completely gone. It was the first time in fifteen years he had been free from the pain.

Another way to help build your confidence is to do good deeds for people. When you do good things for people out of your soul you will have no worries and you will always feel joy in your heart. When you do good things, observe how happy it makes you feel. Try doing them without expecting anything in return and you will find that the more good things you do for people without asking for anything in return, the more good things will return back to you. As more good things return to you, your confidence will continue to grow and you will enjoy doing even more for others.

Call upon the master's energy

Before you practice Spring Forest Qigong active exercises, meditations or use SFQ techniques to help others to heal, call upon your master's energy.

Spring Forest Qigong is energy healing or spiritual healing. We can also think of it as signal healing, informational healing or message healing. We can pass our energy to help others heal, but as an individual we do not have sufficient energy to give. We must draw upon energy outside of our body such as the universal energy and the energy of our master.

Who is the master?

The master is someone who has very purified energy, strong healing energy and for whom you have very high respect. This is a Chinese concept and some people in the west are confused by this.

There are different levels of masters. At the very top, would be a spiritual master, someone of the highest and most purified spiritual energy, such as Jesus Christ, Buddha, Moses or Lao Tzu. At the next level, a master could be someone such as a wonderful and loving grandmother or grandfather. Next would be a teacher such as myself. As you can see, the word master can have many meanings but is always someone for whom you have the highest respect.

To call on your master's energy is easy. Stretch open your hands and call upon your master's energy using the intention of your mind. When you feel a tingly sensation in your hands, warmness runs throughout your body, or you can see light or color around you, or you can smell something very nice and sweet, your master's energy is with you.

If at first you do not have any of those experiences don't be concerned. As you practice and learn to calm your mind and relax yourself you will eventually have the experience of your master's energy and the universal energy flowing into you. Until then, just know and trust that the energy is there and is flowing into you whether you sense it right away or not.

The relationship between you and your master is like the relationship between a radio and radio station. The radio station is constantly sending out a signal and may be broadcasting beautiful, soothing music that you would very much enjoy, but you will not be able to enjoy the music unless you do certain things.

First, you must have your radio turned on. If your radio is off, of course, you won't hear anything, because the radio station is broadcasting but you are not ready to receive the signal.

Secondly, your radio must be tuned to the right station, the right frequency. Sometimes it can take some fine-tuning on your radio to bring in the signal clearly. Yet, once you tune into the right frequency and get the signal, the signal goes through the amplifier and then to the speaker and if the quality of the speaker is good enough, the sound could be so loud and powerful that it makes the whole room shake.

Finally, you must be listening. If you are busy talking or working, your enjoyment of the music will be limited. The music is still there and you can still hear it but to fully enjoy it you must be still, quiet and relaxed. Then, your enjoyment of the beautiful music will be its fullest.

When you call on your master's energy, you are receiving his or her energy signals and this energy has no limits. And so, just as you can never deplete the universal energy, you will never deplete your master's energy. The supply is inexhaustible.

Your respect for your master is just like your radio. It is through your respect that your radio is turned on. The higher your respect and trust for your master or masters the more powerfully you will receive their signal, their energy.

If you do not have respect for your master, you will never be able to tune to the right frequency and receive his signal. So when you call upon a master's energy, call upon that master's energy that you highly respect.

You can call upon more than one master's energy. If you like my energy, you can call upon my energy, as well. But no matter whose energy you call upon, you must have high respect for them. If you call upon someone's energy that you do not truly respect, you will not receive it.

Of course, when you call upon your master's energy, you must do it for a good purpose. The universal energy knows what to do for you. For instance, if you call upon your master's energy to help you heal yourself or others that is great and you will certainly receive it. But, if you call upon your master's energy for something that is selfish or harmful, you will never get it. Your master's energy and the universal energy is pure and to receive it you must be serving a good purpose.

After you call upon your master's energy, trust it. Don't put any doubt into it. Strongly believe that the universal energy will know what should be done. Simply go ahead and do what you are supposed to do. Whatever happens will happen. Whatever is not going to happen will not happen. Trust that what is good and best will happen. It always does.

Visualization

Visualization is a type of energy.

You can enhance your meditation and self-healing with visualization. For example, you might visualize the blockage (kidney/gall stone, bone spur, pain or tumor, or whatever) changing into air or smoke and shooting out of the body. You might visualize a spur as a bird flying out of the body and going back to nature. What you visualize is up to you; simply visualize whatever may help you.

Many years ago there was a gentleman diagnosed with liver cancer. The doctors gave him two months to live. But he said, "I don't want to die. I want to live. I still have so much to do." So, he maintained a healthy diet, exercised and meditated. In his meditation, he visualized hundreds of thousands of dragons flying from the sky and coming into his body. Each dragon took part of the cancer away. Every day he did this for at least two hours. Two years later, he went back to the hospital. The doctors checked him thoroughly. Eventually they were astonished and were able to tell him he was cancer-free.

Visualization is energy. Visualization creates chemical activities in the body. Through those chemical activities we produce the right kind of energy to meet the needs of the body and to help the body open its blockages.

I recommend that you visualize a transparent energy column running up and down the center of the torso to help open the channels in the internal organs. At the same time imagine that with each breath you take you draw energy into every cell of your body, expelling extra, unneeded energy each time you exhale. And, visualize that you are one with the universe, with your body expanding out, reaching to the farthest stars.

Focus

The focus of meditation is different from that of office work. When you focus at your work you have to concentrate very hard on what you are doing. But meditation focus is different. To focus for meditation, bring your energy inside of the body and concentrate on one point, such as your *lower dantian* (which is deep inside behind the belly button.) At the same time use your mind to feel the moving of the energy in all parts of your body. Relax yourself into a state of being so that when you do not focus you feel something and when you do focus the feeling disappears.

When you meditate for your own health or healing, try not to focus on the pain and the sickness. Before you begin you might say in your mind; "I am in the universe. The universe is in my body. The universe and I combine together. All my pain is gone. I am completely healed." Then simply relax yourself. Use your consciousness to feel how wonderful your body is. Feel how healthy you are instead of focusing on what is wrong, because if you focus on what is wrong you might call the pain back.

You might try this little experiment. If you have left shoulder pain, massage your right shoulder, the good one, for ten minutes or so. While you massage the shoulder, feel how good your shoulders are. Ten minutes later, try your left shoulder and see what happens. You may find that your left shoulder feels much better!

So when you practice meditation do not focus on the symptoms, because the symptoms are not the cause of the sickness. If you want to heal yourself you have to go to the root of the sickness. For instance, if a person has a headache we have to find out what is causing the headache. If we only focus on healing in the head we might miss the root cause of the problem and not completely heal the headache. As we know, a headache can have many causes. These can include shoulder pain, chest pain, too much excitement or a blockage in the heel.

One of my clients had been having migraine headaches for ten years and even though she had been to many different doctors and therapists, and tried many different treatments, the headache remained. When I found that the problem was a blockage in her heel I was able to help clear the root of the blockage and since then she has had no more migraine headaches.

So, when you practice qigong, relax. Focus on the feeling of the flowing of the energy. Let go and simply experience what you can feel in your hands, your legs, your face, and the rest of your body. See whether you can feel any heat, tingly sensations or other sensations in the body. Do not look for a particular sensation. Don't expect it. Just relax and allow yourself to experience whatever you do feel. Each person's experience is their own. And each experience you have will likely be different. The sensations may be very strong and powerful or they may be very faint. Simply experience them.

Don't ask how soon you will get healed. Just keep practicing your active exercise and meditation faithfully. The more you can let go in this way, the faster your energy channels will open. If you are too anxious to get well that can form a barrier blocking you from going into the emptiness. In effect, it can cause you to hold onto the blockage instead of letting go. When you can use your focus to relax and let go (instead of to concentrate so hard) you will more easily move into the emptiness and your channels will open much faster.

Consistency

Ideally, qigong exercises and meditation should be practiced everyday, preferably at the same time. In this way you will set up a system of regulation that can be very healthy to the body. If you can, try to practice qigong for at least a half an hour each day. The longer and more consistently you practice, the greater the results will be.

Many people say that they do not have that much time for Qigong. Making time now, however, saves time spent in the doctor's office or at home sick in bed. Qigong practice may also reduce the amount of time needed for sleep. If you do not have half an hour everyday, find twenty minutes, or even ten minutes and soon you will see its benefit and power. Actually with Spring Forest Qigong, you can do an exercise while you are riding in a car, while you are walking, sitting at a concert, waiting at the bus stop or sleeping.

One way to practice focuses on the breath. Simply say in your mind, "I am in the universe. The universe is in my body. The universe and I combine together." Then, focus on your breathing. Take slow, deep breaths. Bring your stomach in a little as you inhale. Let it out a little as you exhale. Feel the healing energy flowing into your body with each breath you take in. Feel any tiredness or pain or sickness, shooting out of your body to the end of the universe every time you breathe out. Fully relax your mind and allow it to go into the emptiness.

The more you practice the greater the benefit. With more practice, the benefits begin to multiply and multiply and multiply. Even a little time spent practicing can be very helpful. Please, don't let a lack of time keep you from experiencing the wonderful healing power of Spring Forest Qigong.

Many people in western culture like to window shop qigong by attending one qigong workshop today, another tomorrow and then next week practicing with another master at another qigong conference. They seem to learn a lot intellectually but do not enjoy the full benefits of qigong. This is not the best way to learn qigong.

Almost all good masters of qigong agree it is best to choose one style of qigong and stay with it for a long time, even the rest of your life. This way you will build up your system and then perhaps one day when you become very good at that style you can explore other qigong styles. Yet, when you shift often from one style to another, you change your regulation system, which makes it very difficult to bring your meditation and your energy to a higher level. Of course, if you haven't found a qigong style that works well for you shop around until you find one.

When you first begin practicing qigong you may feel the energy quite strongly, because in the beginning your body is like a small energy container: only a little energy will fill it up. After you practice for a while, more energy channels in the body open and your body becomes a bigger container. You need more energy to fill it up. When you reach this point you may not feel the energy strongly anymore, yet you have reached the best time to develop your energy further because your body is collecting more energy in order to move to a higher level. If you give up and stop practicing, the already opened channels will close again. Please don't stop. Don't give up. Practice qigong daily and reap the rewards.

The Source of Healing Power and Joy

Quite often people in my class ask me what the source of the healing power of qigong is. The source of qigong healing power is unconditional love, forgiveness and kindness.

The most beautiful aspect of doing qigong is that through healing the body, you learn to understand your life and the freedom of life, both physically and spiritually. You find long- forgotten love, kindness, and forgiveness coming back to you. You feel you have no fears, no struggle, no anger, no hatred, no depression, no worry and no anxiety. The only things left are love, forgiveness and kindness.

People get angry or feel hatred toward each other because they have forgotten their soul. They have forgotten about love and forgiveness. Every person makes mistakes in his or her life. Some are big and some are small. Yet whether we think a friend has made a big mistake or a small mistake, forgive him. Your love energy will help him to heal and give him a chance to learn from his mistake. He will be grateful and when you make a mistake, he may be able to give you the same forgiveness and chance to learn from your mistake in return.

Life is for happiness–the happiness of your family, your community, your country, and the whole world. If life is not for happiness it becomes meaningless. Happiness is not the same as having fun. Having fun may or may not make you happy. Happiness is much greater than this. Happiness is gained by giving your love and forgiveness to others.

Here are four suggestions for true happiness in life:

1. Do more good deeds for others and society.

When you do good things for others your heart fills with joy. This joy is not superficial, but from deep within your heart and soul. When you see your friend happy you see the value of yourself and you find that happiness returns back to you. When you want to do something good for others don't intend to have them do something for you in return in the future. If you do good things for your family, friends and others that you don't even know, without asking for or expecting something in return, but instead simply do it out of your heart, the universe will know and you will be rewarded in the future.

By doing good things for people you help to purify your own energy. The more good things you do for people, the more you can purify yourself.

2. Love people.

When we talk about love, we mean unconditional love, universal love. When you love people you will feel joy to live in the world, whether or not life seems up or down. In this world we have enough stress, worry, struggle and hatred. But we lack love. Only love can heal a wounded soul. Only love can break down the barriers between people. Only love can bring us hope and true happiness. Give your love to others. Share your love with others. Love your family. Love your friends. Love people around you. Love nature. Love the beauty of life. I believe that love is one of the most important reasons that we are here in the world. Through love we purify our energy and find our soul. We all need love and kindness. We do not need fear or jealousy or anger.

As you hold this universal love in your heart and share it with others, you will experience this love returning back to you. This will make you feel even more joyful and because of this, the energy in your body will flow better and blockages in the body will open much faster. I think you have probably heard many stories already in your life about the healing power of love.

3. Forgive others.

When you forgive others, you allow them a chance to purify their energy. You will not lose anything, but you will gain more love and respect from others. Love begets love, forgiveness begets peace, and hatred begets hatred. It can seem very difficult at times to forgive but it is the best thing you can do for yourself.

Often, it is easier to forgive others than to forgive yourself, which is why so many people experience depression. I had a client come to see me. She was a psychologist. Three years after her husband died she found that she had breast cancer. Since her husband had died she had been very depressed and sad because she thought her husband died because she had not taken care of him well enough. Her depression led to blockages that helped to cause her breast cancer.

I did not say too much about it and asked her to close her eyes and meditate. During the healing, her tears kept coming out. Twenty minutes passed and she said she felt much better. Then she set up five more appointments.

When she came back for the second visit she told me that her tumor was smaller and that she felt very grateful. Each time I worked on her, she cried. In the fifth visit she said the tumor had gotten much smaller and was now as small as half a penny. She was very happy about that. When we finished the healing, she was so emotional that she started telling me about her life.

She said that she felt so guilty for not taking good care of her husband when he was sick. He died very quickly after becoming ill. It was only after her husband passed away that she realized how much she had loved him. She felt she could not live without him.

She cried everyday and became very depressed. Whenever she was alone, she could not help thinking of her husband. She felt so guilty, blamed herself and had no hope in her life. Then, one day when she found a lump in her right breast she was so frightened. She went to the doctor and the tests showed it was cancer.

We chatted quite a bit. At the end of our conversation, I said, "You are a psychologist. I am sure that you know how much our emotions affect our bodies, so let me ask you a question. Everyday you work so hard. For what?" she looked at me and asked back, "What do you think?" I said, "For survival?" "Right." She agreed.

"In order to survive, we do all kinds of things to make sure that our life is protected. We want the best insurance we can get. We want the safest place to live in and the best vehicle to drive. If life is for survival what kind of quality of life are we surviving for; happiness or sadness?" "Happiness, of course." She answered.

"Then where can we find happiness? Can we find happiness in the grief of the past? Of course not. No matter how sad you are, the fact is that your husband has already moved on in his circle of life. Your sadness, depression and tears will never help to bring his life back to you. But, it can affect your survival."

"You cannot undo what is already done. If you really think that you owe your husband something, why not use this as a lesson? In the future you will know how to take better care of your family and friends and you will be inspired to do more good deeds for the people around you. Your husband will watch you in heaven and when he sees this he will be very happy for you and very proud of you."

"Throw the heavy sack full of junk stuff on your back away. Look for your happiness today. I think happiness is waiting for you and if you understand what I mean, you don't need to come back to see me. We can cancel your last appointment. Your blockage will go away by itself."

She looked at me and said that she had never thought in this way. She said that she would think about what I said. One week later, she came back to see me. She said that she was going to throw the heavy sack on her back away and live a happy life, but had wanted to come back to see me because she liked my energy.

I never saw Nancy again but a couple of years later a woman came to visit me and said Nancy wanted her to say hi to me. It had been so long I did not remember who Nancy was until she reminded me. When I asked how Nancy was doing she told me that Nancy was doing fine and that her tumor had been gone for over two years, ever since my last appointment with her. She was a very happy and healthy lady now.

Nancy had been healthy all her life but after her husband died she was so weighted down with guilt that it created great stress and depression. The "weight" of those emotions contributed to her illness by creating many energy blockages in her body that kept her energy from being balanced.

By using Spring Forest Qigong healing techniques I was able to remove the blockages and help restore her energy balance. But, if Nancy had kept carrying that "heavy sack of junk" around, the blockages would have returned.

People often tend to remember the bad times more than the happy times. For example, when a friend has done something that has hurt us terribly we might forget all of the good memories and only focus on the hurt, anger or sadness. Our friend may also feel sad, angry or guilty, perhaps even for the rest of his life. This is a passive way to deal with our emotions and leads to depression and sickness. If depression, hurt feelings and anger are not things that we want, why not put them away and replace them with forgiveness?

We cannot change the past but we can choose to learn from it – forgive – and move on to enjoy a happy life.

4. The fourth suggestion: Be flexible.

Do not be so stubborn. We are living in a changing world. Opportunities come our way and then pass by us every day. Concepts change from day to day and what is in fashion today can become history tomorrow. Life has no fixed patterns. If you want to eat a potato for dinner today but you do not have it on hand find something else. Why go hungry or spoil your dinnertime being irritated? Be a flexible person and you will find it easier and more enjoyable to deal with things around you.

Another important reason for us to be flexible is that everything has its own cycle. What is going to happen will happen and what is not going to happen will not happen. Anxiety, stress and depression are some of the greatest causes of energy blockages in the body. Why do people have these things? I think there are two main reasons:

First, as human beings we often want something to happen when we want it to happen even if it is not the right time for us. I think most of us agree that everyone has their own purpose and potential in life. No two people in the world are exactly the same. Yet many of us have a desire that, for instance, when we are twenty years old we experience something such as fame and that we will be wealthy when we are forty. Even if it is not right for us and not aligned with our potential at that particular time, we may push too hard and force ourselves to reach the goal. We may put too much pressure on ourselves and when we do not achieve what we want, develop anxiety, stress and depression. Not surprisingly, even if we do achieve what we were so fiercely striving for, we may find it wasn't what we wanted after all and still feel unhappy.

Secondly, we may compare our life to another's and feel jealous. An example could be someone who is a struggling actor comparing themselves to another person who has become a famous international movie star. He may complain, "I have the same talents or even more than he does. Why is he a famous movie star and not me? That is not fair." This way of thinking can develop into jealousy, and later on the jealousy can develop into anxiety, stress and depression.

In truth, we all know everyone has her and his own special way to contribute to the beauty of the world. In the world things are not positive or negative until we think of them as positive or negative. Why not just take everything easy? Be still and follow your inner voice to do whatever you are asked to do. Take everything that happens as a great opportunity to help you to grow. After all, what looks like a positive thing can turn out to be a negative thing and a negative thing can turn out to be a positive thing.

For instance, in Shakespeare's time, the word "N-I-C-E" meant something foolish or stupid. But now it means something good, very comforting. Well, no matter if it was in the past or in the modern time, it is still the same four letters and spells the same thing. Over time we simply changed the meaning and what was once negative is now positive.

So practice taking things easy. Whatever will be will be. There is no need to judge. As long as you know you are doing good things for people, no matter what other people may think or say about you, simply continue with what you are doing. If you do this you will find peace in your mind and you will live a happy life.

Qigong has been practiced in China for many millennia but is still new in western culture. As I have mentioned before, some people who do not understand what qigong is, compare it to a religion. As a Spring Forest Qigong practitioner you may need to explain patiently to your family that qigong is not religion. It is a study of the human body and actually is a science which has nothing to do with religion.

Of course, qigong is a spiritual practice in that we are all spiritual beings. We are not just flesh and blood. We are much more than that. We each have an eternal soul and the power of qigong flows from the love, kindness and forgiveness in our soul. I have studied with many great qigong masters and while they taught very different techniques they all shared this in common. Each of these qigong masters taught that the power of qigong comes from love, kindness and forgiveness. The universal energy flows through the love, kindness and forgiveness we have in our soul and without an awareness of those things we cannot experience the full beauty and benefits of qigong.

If your family or friends do not accept this, do not force it on them. Allow them more time. Show them the scientific studies on qigong or buy them one of the many qigong books available. Send them love energy. If they are open to trying qigong teach them one or two of the exercises and let them experience the power and the beauty of qigong for themselves. Believe that if it is meant to be, eventually they will open their minds and hearts and become a qigong practitioner, too.

I have a student who has become a very good Qigong practitioner, but when she first came to my class her husband was not very happy. She felt so sad about this that she cried in class. We comforted her, and her very close relatives also supported her, saying that they believed some day her husband would understand what she was doing. One night her husband had a bad stomach ache. He tried everything in the house, but nothing worked. Eventually he woke his wife up and said, "Do you want to try your thing on me?" "What thing?" she asked. "The thing you practice everyday." She sent energy to help remove the blockage – and the pain went away! Now he has referred many of his friends to his wife and he himself practices qigong.

So, when you meet with difficulty, don't argue. Don't struggle. Be loving and forgiving. Que sera, sera. Whatever will be will be. When it is time it is time. You can never control what others think or say or do. You can only be the best example of what you believe.

Practice your Qigong today, be happy and focus on the beauty of life.

Spring Forest Qigong

Exercises & Meditations

春林氣功

Part One: Active Exercises

Main Benefits of Exercises

The active exercises are like moving meditations. They strengthen our physical energy and help to open all of the energy channels in the body. They help bring our Yin and Yang energy back into balance, get rid of energy blockages and develop our spiritual energy so that we can heal physically, mentally and spiritually at the same time.

When doing the active exercises without the CD or DVD for guidance you can do any combination of the individual exercises for any amount of time. Also, you can practice these exercises while standing, sitting or lying down. (Remember: good, better, best and simply do the best that you can, knowing you will receive the benefit you need.) Spring Forest Qigong Level One active exercises open all the energy channels in the body through gentle movement and helping to focus the mind and breath. Try doing the active exercises at least once daily.

The level one series consists of the following exercises which are described in detail on the following pages:

1.   **Beginning of the Universe**

2.   **Forming of Yin and Yang**

3.   **Moving of Yin and Yang**

4.   **Breathing of the Universe**

5.   **Joining of Yin and Yang**

6.   **Harmony of Universal Energy**

7.   **Seven Steps of New Life**

8.   **Ending: Harvesting of Qi**

1 - Beginning of the Universe

This exercise brings your focus back into your body and wakes up the internal energy.

Time on CD and DVD: 2 to 3 minutes

Time to practice on your own: 2 to 3 minutes or longer if you wish

There are many energy channels in the body, but the most important ones are the front channel and the back channel. The front channel runs through the front and middle of the body; the back channel runs along the spine to the head.

All the other channels work around these two channels and so a blockage in these two channels will result in a problem in the body. When you practice this exercise, place your tongue against the roof of your mouth, because the tongue acts as the switch connecting the two channels.

When practicing this exercise you may notice tingling sensations in your fingers and feet as the energy channels in the feet and the hands wake up.

It is a good idea to do "Beginning of the Universe" for 2 – 3 minutes prior to practicing any of the other SFQ active exercises. This will help you to become more settled, more aware of your body and breath and more connected with the universal energy.

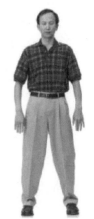

- When doing this exercise standing, stand straight, toes pointing forward, knees slightly bent.

- Set your feet a little more than shoulder width apart for good balance.

- Wear a smile on your face to relax every part of the body and stimulate the brain

to produce endorphins.

- Draw your chin back a little to straighten the entire spine. (Energy travels up and down the spine in the governing channel more easily when the spine is straight.)

- Gaze forward and close your eyes.

- Gently rest the tip of your tongue on the roof of your mouth.

- Open your fingers.

- Drop the shoulders. Gently hold the elbows outward.

- Slowly take a deep, silent and gentle breath through your nose. As you breathe in, draw the lower part of your stomach in a little. As you breathe out, let your stomach out.

- Imagine using your whole body to breathe. Visualize the universal energy coming into every cell of your body and collecting in the lower dantian. (The lower dantian is the body's primary energy center located deep behind the navel.)

- When you exhale, visualize any pain or sickness changing into smoke and shooting out from every cell of your body to the end of the universe.

- Gently say in your mind:

"I am in the universe.
The universe is in my body.
The universe and I combine together."

- Feel the emptiness, quietness, and stillness of the universe.

2 - Forming of Yin & Yang

Hold this posture to rebalance the energy in the body.

Time on CD and DVD: 3 minutes
Time to practice on your own: 3 to 5 minutes or longer if you wish

The upper part of the torso above the navel belongs to Yang energy and the lower part of the torso under the navel belongs to Yin energy. One of the reasons people get sick is because the Yin-Yang energies scatter and are not in good balance. This exercise helps to balance those energies.

When doing this exercise you may feel tingly sensations in your hands and warmth in the chest and lower stomach, which are areas faced by your palms. You may also feel a current running in the middle of the torso or along the spine, which is the energy channels opening.

- To begin, slowly raise your right hand (the Yang male energy) to the upper chest and your left hand (the Yin female energy) to the lower stomach. Your palms face your body, without touching it, to create a sensation of emptiness.

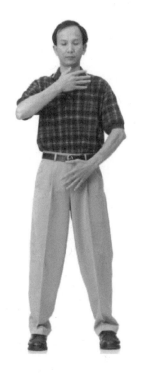

- Visualize a transparent energy column in the middle of your torso shining with beautiful colors. The energy column runs from the head to the bottom of the torso and can be larger or smaller depending upon your visualization.

- As you hold your hands in this posture drop your elbows and remain still so that energy flows uninterrupted.

- Continue to feel the emptiness of the universe as you remain in this position.

3 - Moving of Yin & Yang

This exercise is the fundamental exercise of SFQ. It balances and helps heal all the internal organs, opens the heart and aligns the spine.

Time on CD and DVD: 13 minutes
Time to practice on your own: 10 to 60 minutes

During this exercise the palms face the central line of the torso where there are lots of energy points related to the internal organs. Through the guidance of your mind and the movement of your hands the heart energy and the kidney energy join. Blockages open.

- Stand with your feet a little more than shoulder width apart, toes pointed forward, knees slightly bent. Wear a smile on your face. Draw your chin back to straighten the spine. Relax and drop the shoulders. Open your fingers.

- Begin in the "Forming of Yin and Yang" posture. When you are settled begin to move your hands. Your right hand moves out and down to the bottom of the torso while your left hand moves in and up to your face. Your hands continue moving in this circular pattern

- Visualize a transparent energy column of beautiful colors running from the top of the head to the bottom of the torso. While moving the hands, visualize the energy moving up and down the transparent column. Imagine the channels in the torso opening completely.

- *Feel the energy.* Use your elbows to guide the movements and use your hands to feel the energy.

- Move your hands as slowly as possible (3 – 5 circles per minute to begin). Moving more slowly = more energy.

- As you continue the movement, try to keep your fingers open in order to better receive energy.

Tip: Try not to move your spine from side to side, because that movement interferes with your energy moving deeper into the emptiness level.

4 - Breathing of the Universe

This exercise heals the lungs and skin and balances the energy inside and outside of the body.

> *Time on CD and DVD: 6 minutes*
> *Time to practice on your own: 6 to 30 minutes*

During this exercise the movement of your hands combined with the breathing technique helps to open blockages in the whole body, especially the lungs.

As you practice try to feel the energy as it expands in the space between your hands as you open them and then compresses as you close them. Your hands do not touch each other.

- Begin with both hands facing each other in front of the *lower dantian* (navel area.)

- Keep a space between the body and the hands and between both hands. In this way you can keep the feeling of emptiness.

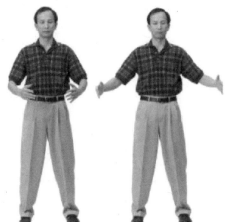

- With your awareness in your lower dantian take three deep breaths.

- Then, as you inhale move your hands open to the sides; exhale as you close your hands.

- Use your hands and body to feel the energy while you use the elbows to guide the action. (Your hands do not touch.)

- Use your whole body to breathe. While you inhale, visualize the pure universal energy flowing into your body from every part of the body and gathering in the lower dantian.

- While you exhale, imagine any sickness or pain turning into air or smoke and shooting out from every part of the body to the end of the universe.

- Stay still and relaxed. Gently rest your tongue against the roof of your mouth. Wear a smile.

5 - Joining of Yin and Yang

This exercise balances the energy in the body.

Time on CD and DVD: 6 minutes
Time to practice on your own: 6 to 30 minutes

As you practice this exercise you build energy in the *lower dantian* (the energy center deep behind the navel.)

- Begin with both hands facing each other in front of the *lower dantian* as in the previous exercise (Breathing of the Universe)

- Imagine your hands coming together around a ball of energy about the size of a volleyball.

- Imagine you are in that ball of energy.

- Keep your fingers open so the energy can flow.

- Keep your palms facing each other.

- Begin "rolling the ball" by moving your hands from top to bottom and from bottom to top.

- Move slowly feeling the energy.

- Continue rolling the ball.

- Imagine your body's energy is in the ball and is being totally renewed.

6 - Harmony of the Universe

This exercise helps to open blockages, heal the body, and balance the energy in the left and right brain. It also helps move your spiritual energy to a higher level.

Time on CD and DVD: 15 minutes
Time to practice on your own: 15 to 30 minute, or longer

During this exercise, as you move your hands and body you open blockages in the lungs, breasts, liver, spine, shoulders, lower back and hips. When you practice this exercise with your eyes closed you may see more colors.

1. Receive energy from the universe with your hands.

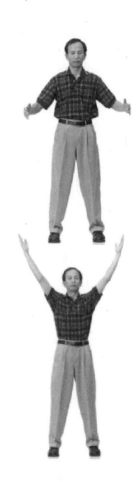

2. As you inhale, raise the energy ball up in front of you and up over your head. Open your hands and arms wide above your head, palms up, head slightly up.

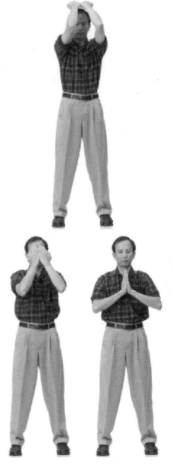

3. Hold your breath as you bring your hands together, closing your fingers. Bring the energy down with your hands to cover your head without touching your head. Hold for three seconds.

4. Exhale as you bring your hands down, passing the face. As you reach the chin, bring your hands together, palms in and continue moving your hands down until you come to your lower stomach.

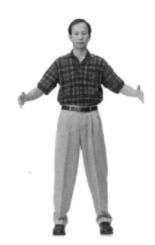

5. Inhale. Open your fingers as you open your hands wide to the sides as you did in "Breathing of the Universe." Use your elbows to guide the movement and your hands to feel the energy

6. Exhale as you bring your hands in, collecting more energy.

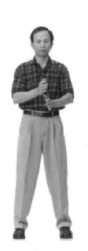

7. Keep closing your hands until they pass each other and are in line with the elbow area with your right hand on top first and left hand at the bottom. Your palms face down; hands do not touch the elbows.

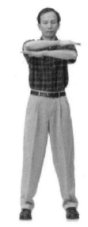

8. Inhale; lower your head down and lean forward to the right until your head is over the right elbow without touching the elbow. Your head turns slightly to the left. Remain in this position as you exhale.

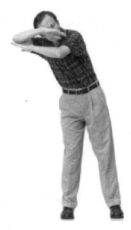

9. Inhale, drawing the right hand up and to the right until your arm is straight. The fingers of the right hand continue pointing to the left with the palm facing down. At the same time, your left hand moves out pressing down to the left.

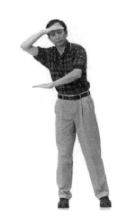

10. Fingers point to the right with the palm down. (This opens all six energy channels in your hands. If you turn your fingers outward, only three channels open.) Lean forward to the right as you raise your left heel up pointing the toes. (Moving the heels up and down can help open the six channels in the feet.)

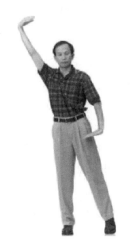

11. Exhale as you open the right hand, turn it facing down and smoothly move it down in a circle, as the left hand moves in until you are holding the energy ball between your hands once again.

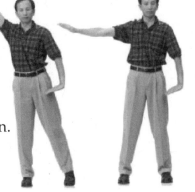

12. Repeat the cycle, this time moving to your left (for step 8). Alternate right and left with each cycle and end on the opposite side you began.

7 - Seven Steps of New Life

This exercise helps to improve balance and heal the body. It is especially helpful for arthritis, cold hands and cold feet.

Time on CD and DVD: 10 minutes
Time to practice on your own: 10 to 30 minutes

This is the "plunger" technique. Like a bellows, you draw energy into the body, collect it in your lower dantian and pump it throughout the entire body. This exercise opens and clears all of the body's energy channels.

Starting with your left leg, imagine using your whole body as a bellows for moving energy to these seven levels:

1 — Navel

2 — Heart

3 — Shoulders

4 — Throat

5 — Nose

6 — Forehead

7 — Top of the Head

(Warning: Pregnant women should skip this exercise. The movement of the energy might disturb the peace of the baby. It will not harm the baby but is not helpful.)

Seven Steps of New Life (continued)

- Inhale and visualize universal energy flowing into your body through every cell and collecting in the first level behind the navel.

- Exhale, pushing the energy down to the toes.

- Inhale again, drawing the energy from the toes up to the second level, the heart level.

- Exhale, pushing the energy down to the toes.

- Repeat this process multiple times through all of the levels.

Use your hands to guide the energy. On each inhale, move your hands up to the upper chest with your palms facing up. On each exhale, move your hands down to your lower torso with your palms facing down.

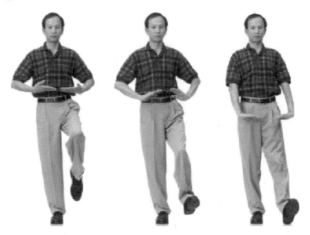

On each inhale, lift your leg with the toes pointing to the ground. On each exhale, step forward to press your heel to the ground. Always start with your left leg and alternate through the exercise.

You may do as many rounds of the seven levels as you wish. When finished, inhale one more time. Visualize energy flowing into your body and collecting in your lower dantian. Exhale without focusing your mind on anything.

8 – Ending Exercises: Harvesting of Qi

These exercises balance and adjust the energy in the body and help the body to heal faster.

Time on CD and DVD: 10 minutes
Time to practice on your own: 10 minutes

Each of the SFQ Active Exercises (1 – 7) can be practiced separately. You might choose one or two movements each day or you might choose to do them all. However, always finish with the ending exercises. This will bring you out of your meditation and help put the *Qi* into the right places of your body.

Also, when you choose to do active exercises and a sitting meditation together, do the active exercises first in order to make it easier to go into the emptiness. Then follow the sitting meditation with the ending exercises.

1. Rub your hands together, palm to palm.

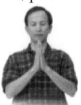

2. Massage your face: with your palms toward your face use your middle fingers to push up along the bridge of the nose until your fingers reach the forehead; cover the face with your hands; and part your hands as they draw down the face to the chin.

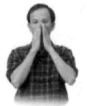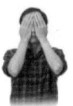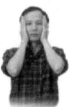

3. Comb your head with your fingers from front to the back of the head. The tips of your fingers touch your scalp.

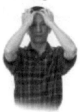

4. Form your hands into a cup. Pat your head with your cupped hands from front to back.

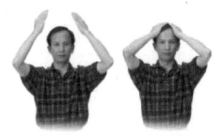

5. Massage your ears from top to bottom. Massage every part of the ear.

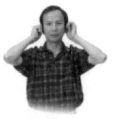

6. Cup your hands again and pat the inside and outside of each arm.

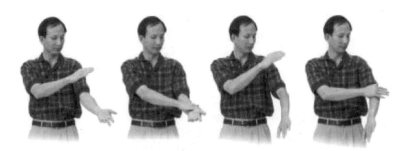

7. Pat the chest and stomach from top to bottom.

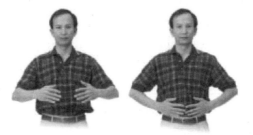

8. Pat the underarm area on the left side and then the right side.

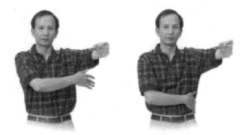

9. Massage the stomach by interlacing your fingers and massage right to left in a clockwise direction.

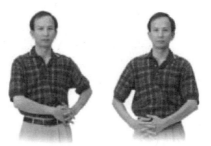

10. Bend over at the waist. Cup your hands again and pat the kidney area. Then, use the back of your hands to massage this area several times. Turn your hands over and massage the kidneys a few more times.

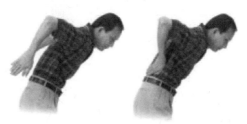

11. Tapping the Tailbone (not pictured): Remain bent over, lean your head and neck forward so that there is a slight curve to your spine. Pat the tailbone and sacrum area with cupped hands or loose fists for two or three minutes. The tailbone is the gate of vitality in the body. Tapping the tailbone strengthens the kidney energy and balances energy that helps with weight control, reproductive problems, fertility, headaches and memory.

12. Support your kidneys by covering them with your hands and slowly straighten the body by lifting the back and shoulders. Lift the head last.

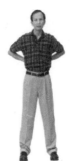

13. Use your chin to draw a horizontal circle from left to right six to nine times. Repeat in the other direction.

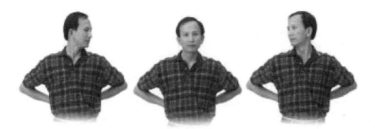

14. Dolphin the neck by moving the head slightly forward and up, then down and back. This is the same as drawing a vertical circle. Do this six to nine times.

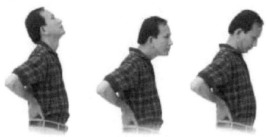

15. Support the kidney area with your hands and dolphin the whole spine: move the upper part of the body forward first; bend the knees and move the knees forward; and extend the stomach, the chest, and the head. Do this six to nine times.

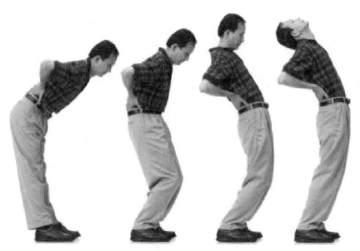

16. Straighten the body. Lift your hands up in front of your chest with your palms down and your elbows slightly higher than the shoulders. Look forward. Lead with the elbows and swing your arms from left to right, keeping your head and hips facing forward. Do this six to nine times.

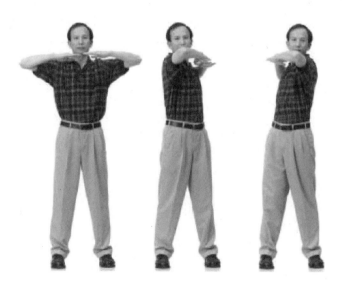

17. Lower the elbows to the stomach level and repeat the swing motion six to nine times. (Be gentle if you have severe lower back problems.)

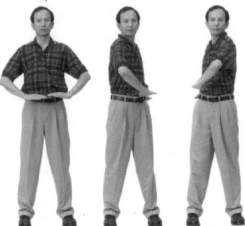

18. Tapping of Hip Points (not pictured): Form your hands into soft fists again and tap the hips. The area you want to tap is behind the top of the leg bone and below the pelvic girdle. It's in the area where you'll find a dimple or impression on the side of the buttocks. Pat for 1 or 2 minutes.

19. Rest your hands down at your sides. Lift your body up by stretching the heels up (that is, standing on your toes) and dropping the heels down six to nine times.

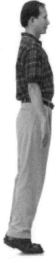

(Note: Pregnant women should skip this heel drop exercise.)

Active Exercises – Addendum

In the ending exercises we have movements that involve the spine and massaging and patting the body. Let's explore why we do these exercises.

Massaging the hands

There are six main channels starting from the fingers. Two heart channels start from the middle and the little fingers. The lung channel starts from the thumb. The large intestine channel starts from the index finger. The small intestine channel starts from the little finger. The pancreas channel starts from the ring finger. When we massage the hands and the insides of the fingers it helps to open those important energy channels.

Massaging the face and ears

The face and ears have points linking to energy channels in all parts of the body. And so, when you massage your face and ears you massage your whole body. For example, if you feel pain when you massage your ears you have a blockage in the relative part or organ in the body. Keep massaging that point on your ear until the pain is completely gone – the blockage in the body will disappear.

Massaging the kidneys

Kidney energy is the most important energy for our life and vitality. If we use up our kidney energy too fast our lives will end sooner. A man's kidney energy begins to decrease after age 40 and a woman's after age 35. Our legs are the first parts of the body to indicate we are aging. When we feel our legs are not as strong as before our kidney energy is getting lower. In Tao meditation, Chinese medicine and longevity exercises, the kidney energy is always number one in our attention. When we massage our kidneys we help energize and balance this vital energy center.

Cupping exercise

The areas to be cupped have almost all of the energy channels. Cupping wakes up and moves the energy in those channels and clears away blockages. (Note: If you catch a cold, cup your arms to help stop coughing, because the lung, heart, and large intestine channels run through the arms.)

Spine exercise

Most human ailments relate to blockages in the spine. Mental problems and other sickness in the head relate to the neck. Illnesses in the major organs relate to the back spine. Reproductive organ problems relate to the lower back and the tailbone. The spine exercises balance and energize that vitally important area of the body.

Patting the Tailbone

The tailbone is the gate of vitality in the body. Tapping the tailbone strengthens the kidney energy and balances energy that helps with weight control, reproductive problems, fertility, headaches and memory.

Getting up every couple of hours to pat the tailbone and sacrum area will help open channels that have closed due to long periods of sitting or other blockages. Also, SFQ recommends that women over 35 spend several minutes patting the tailbone area every day to prevent blockages in the female organs.

Heel exercise

When you move the heels up and down you open the energy channels in your feet including the liver and kidney channels. This exercise is very good for constipation as well as cold feet and hands in the wintertime.

Walking and running exercise

When you walk or run, put your tongue against the roof of the mouth. Swing your hands naturally from side to side with your fingers open and form a Yin-Yang circle. Visualize or imagine you are walking or running in the sun.

As you inhale, imagine the pure universal energy running into the body through every cell and gathering deep in behind the navel. As you exhale, imagine any sickness and all energy blockages change into smoky air and shoot out from every cell to the end of the universe. These exercises can be done any time.

Sleeping exercise

Put your tongue against the roof of the mouth. Inhale and exhale the same as walking and running exercises. You can sleep on your back or on either side. Do not sleep on your stomach, because your neck will twist and blockages can gradually develop.

Visualize you are sleeping in the moon. Before you fall asleep, say to yourself: "May I sleep for eight hours in eight hours of Qigong meditation. Tomorrow, when I wake-up, all my energy channels are open. I have no energy blockages in my body. I am completely healed."

Before getting out of bed first thing in the morning take a deep breath three times, rub your hands, and massage your face.

This exercise is especially useful for those who have sleeping problems.

Part Three: Sitting Meditations

The sitting meditations open energy channels by developing mental concentration and controlled breathing.

In Level One of Spring Forest Qigong we practice two sitting meditations. The sitting meditations use mental concentration, controlled breathing and sound to open the front and back energy channels.

The Small Universe is the sitting meditation most often recommended and is available alone or as part of several different SFQ products.

The Self-Concentration meditation can only be found in the *Level One for Health Sitting Meditations CD*, which includes both of these sitting meditations.

To begin either meditation, sit in a chair with your spine straight and feet flat on the floor. Place your hands over your knees with your palms up. (If you have high blood pressure, place your hands in your lap with your palms down.) Keep your fingers extended to prevent falling asleep.

Small Universe

This meditation helps to clear energy blockages along the two most important channels in the body, the front and back channels.

Time on CD: 30 minutes (Level One Sitting Meditations CD), or
30 minutes or 60 minutes (Small Universe CD)
Time to practice on your own: 30 minutes to 1 hour

We have many energy channels and energy centers in our bodies. When energy starts at one point, visits all the channels and centers in the body, and comes back to the starting point, we have what is literally translated from Chinese ancient wisdom as a "big universe."

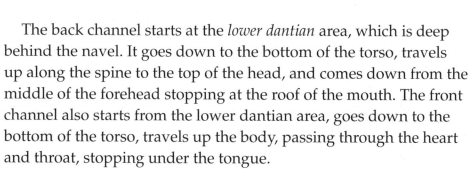

The most important channels are the back and front channels in the torso. When energy starts at one point on those channels, visits all the parts of the system, and comes back to the starting point, we have what is called a "small universe." Many small universes make up a big universe.

The back channel starts at the *lower dantian* area, which is deep behind the navel. It goes down to the bottom of the torso, travels up along the spine to the top of the head, and comes down from the middle of the forehead stopping at the roof of the mouth. The front channel also starts from the lower dantian area, goes down to the bottom of the torso, travels up the body, passing through the heart and throat, stopping under the tongue.

These two channels control and influence the other channels in the body. They automatically connect together four hours a day: at noon from 11:00 am to 1:00 pm and at midnight from 11:00 pm to 1:00 am. Qigong practitioners like to meditate at midnight and at noon, because it takes less energy and generates greater benefits.

Nearly all of the important energy centers are arranged along the back and front channels. As a result, a blockage in the heart energy center could cause heart, lung, breast, chest, or intelligence problems. A blockage in the tailbone could cause reproductive organ problems, low sexual energy, and headaches. A blockage in the cervical bone #7 of the spinal cord could cause headaches, fever, diabetes, and lung and heart problems.

The Small Universe is the easiest meditation technique to open these two channels:

- Concentrate your mind in the *lower dantian* (behind the navel).

- Visualize your own energy and all your generational energy (the energy automatically passed down from generation to generation) joining together, shining very brightly in your *lower dantian.*

- Listen to the master's voice on the CD. You'll hear two sounds [... O O H M ...] and [... M U A H...].

- These sounds are extremely powerful, because their vibration can reach every corner of the body to clear blockages. Each time you hear the sound inhale, and then, in between the sounds exhale.

- On each inhale, visualize the master's energy and the universal energy joining together and radiating into an area of your body.

- On each exhale, move the energy to the next area of your body. The specific areas of your body are shown in the photograph below.

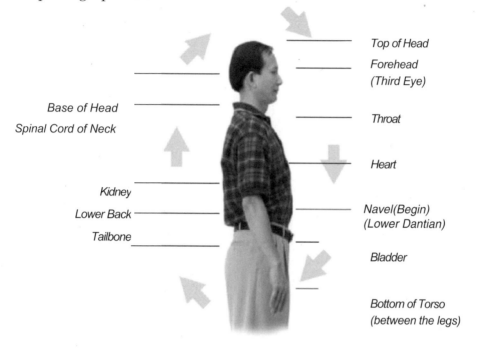

Top of Head

Forehead
(Third Eye)

Base of Head
Spinal Cord of Neck

Throat

Heart

Kidney
Lower Back
Tailbone

Navel(Begin)
(Lower Dantian)

Bladder

Bottom of Torso
(between the legs)

- Then start all over again from the *lower dantian*.

- You can continue to move the energy through the Small Universe for as many rounds as you want. But when you are finished stop at the *lower dantian*. Visualize the energy as a ball moving clockwise inside the *lower dantian*. The energy ball gets smaller and smaller, finally changing into an energy pill that hides deep in behind the navel. When finished, take a deep breath three times. Rub your hands. Finish with the ending exercises.

Self-Concentration

This guided meditation helps heal the body and develop personal self-awareness.

Time on CD: 30 minutes
Time to do on your own: 30 minutes to 1 hour

By using mental concentration and controlled breathing you move to a deeper level of meditation.

- Listen to the CD and simply follow along.

- Wear a smile on your face.

- Take three deep breaths, inhaling through your nose and exhaling through your mouth to clear away toxins in the stomach.

- Say in your mind the password:

"I am in the universe.

The universe is in my body.

The universe and I combine together."

- Say in your mind:

"All my channels open, open, open, completely open.

I have no energy blockages in my body.

All my pain is gone.

I am completely healed."

- Feel your whole spine, starting from the tailbone, growing longer, straighter, longer, straighter, even straighter, completely straight.

- Feel all the channels within your body open: the head channels, the neck channels, the shoulder channels, the chest channels, the back channels, the stomach channels, the lower back channels, the tailbone channels, the channels in the bottom of the torso, the thigh channels, the leg channels, and the feet channels.

- Feel any blockages in the lungs, liver, and pancreas change into smoke and disappear. Any stones within the body explode and turn into smoke and disappear. Any tumors within the body turn into smoke and completely disappear. Visualize the inside of your body as clean and healthy.

- Imagine that you are in the season of spring as a happy little girl or boy, running on the green grass. The air is fresh, sun warm, trees green, water blue, and flowers beautiful. Birds sing sweetly. Children play. You have no worry, sadness, sorrow, depression, or stress. You feel safe, peaceful, and relaxed. Burdens are gone. Love, kindness and forgiveness are all coming back to you. You feel happy and healthy, totally lost in the harmony of the universe.

- When finished, take a deep breath three times. Rub your hands. Massage your face. Cup your head. Massage your ears.

Helpful Tips

I recommend that you do the Active Exercises, any component of the Active Exercises, or one of the meditations at least twice a week for one hour. I strongly recommend that you do the exercises or meditations at least once a day. You will receive more benefit if you do it three times each day, especially for those people who may have severe blockages in the body.

The best time for exercise and meditation is whenever you can fit them into your schedule. Beyond that we find the best times for doing the Active Exercises are in the morning and early in the evening. The best times for the Sitting Meditations are in the morning, at noon, and in the late evening around midnight, because the energy during these times is more balanced.

The following are some additional tips for practicing Spring Forest Qigong. However, please keep in mind that there is no right or wrong in SFQ – only "good, better and best." Trust your inner guidance to show you what is best for you right now, knowing that as long as you continue to practice you will receive benefit.

- Find a quiet place free of distractions such as the telephone.

- Wear comfortable clothes that do not constrict the body.

- When practicing the active exercises move your hands and legs as slowly as possible. The slower, the better. This will allow you to feel the energy better and more easily experience the emptiness.

- If possible do not eat 30 minutes before or after the qigong exercise, because the digestion process may absorb energy that otherwise would be used for healing.

- Try not to have anything cold to drink 30 minutes before you practice qigong, because cold energy can interfere with the flowing of the *Qi*.

- Although there are no maximum time limits for any of the exercises, you may want to take a break during sessions lasting more than two hours.

- If you are too excited or too emotional it is difficult to focus, quiet the mind, and go into the emptiness. Try to settle yourself down before you begin your exercise or wait until you are not so emotional.

- If possible do not use the bathroom within 30 minutes after the exercise because this can cause you to lose *Qi*. (If it is not possible to wait, try bringing your awareness to your heart center and gently lifting your heels up as you use the bathroom. This will help keep the healing energy in the body.)

- Avoid using alcohol before or after practicing qigong because alcohol depletes *Qi* and affects the mind.

- Avoid exercising during a thunderstorm, because the storm makes it difficult to go into the emptiness. Also, do not practice outside in the rain, wind or snow.

- Avoid washing your hands or face with cold water or taking a bath immediately after your qigong practice because this can deplete *Qi* and can even make you ill.

- As much as possible follow the instructions contained in this Spring Forest Qigong Personal Learning Course.

- Avoid mixing Spring Forest Qigong movements with other energy techniques.

- Finally, please get the advice of a medical doctor before

beginning this or any other exercise program. This is particularly important if you have a health concern.

Experiences and sensations while practicing Spring Forest Qigong can include:

- Tingling sensations

- Seeing colors and images

- Itching on your body

- Smelling something sweet like incense or lotus flowers – this is your master's energy or spiritual energy coming to help you

- The sensation of a breeze

- Sensations of heat inside your body

- A feeling of electricity flowing through your body

- Hearing unknown sounds

- Automatic movement of the body

- Crying or tearing

- Feeling sadness (When this sadness is not for something specific, but is for the whole universe, this means your soul energy has awakened. This is a very powerful healing energy.)

- The pain or the symptoms worsening. (This can happen as we are releasing and rebalancing energy blockages, especially for those who have arthritis or structural damage after accidents. The pain usually does not stay long and is an indication that energy is trying to heal and bring the body to its normal condition. Only ten percent of people who have arthritis or structural problems experience more pain. When this happens, please call your doctor for advice before continuing the exercise.)

Any or none of those experiences can occur while practicing Spring Forest Qigong, however it is helpful to take it easy and not be too concerned or go looking for any particular experience during our SFQ practice. We can trust that whatever occurs is just what we need to help release blockages and rebalance our energy at that particular time.

Additional resources

At Spring Forest Qigong, our mission is to provide you with the knowledge, techniques, support and assistance to awaken the natural healing ability you were born with.   We do this by offering:

- Classes and Retreats
- Individual Sessions
- Coaching
- Home Study
- Instructional DVD's and CD's
- Meditation CD's
- Workshops and Conferences

SFQ will help you achieve optimal health, wellness and fitness, and live a life without pain.

To learn more about Spring Forest Qigong please visit our websites at:
www.springforestqigong.com or **www. bornahealer.com**

"A healer in every family
and a world without pain"

SFQ

FUNDAMENTALS

SUGGESTED INSTRUCTIONS

SFQ Fundamentals introduces you to the basics of **Spring Forest Qigong**, including SFQ Active Exercises and the Small Universe. These simple yet powerful tools utilize breath, visualization, sound, and simple movements to help you relax completely and heal physically, mentally, and spiritually. Anyone and everyone—regardless of ability, age, or beliefs—can practice the techniques of SFQ.

TO BEGIN:

1) Familiarize yourself with the manual that is included. You can use this as a reference to assist you as you learn SFQ.

2) Watch the DVD and follow along with the simple, powerful movements of the SFQ Active Exercises.

3) For the Small Universe meditation, simply sit, or lie comfortably, play the CD, and follow along as Master Chunyi Lin guides you through this powerful meditation.

We have found, as in any practice, the more you use these techniques, the more benefit you will receive. In Spring Forest Qigong there is no right or wrong way to practice—only good, better, and best.

To learn more about Spring Forest Qigong please visit our websites at:
www.springforestqigong.com